Wisdom for My Daughters

Wisdom for My Daughters

Melissa Dugan

Publisher: Dugan Publishing

ISBN: 979-8-9948641-0-4 (Hardcover)

ISBN: 979-8-9948641-1-1 (Paperback)

ISBN: 979-8-9948641-2-8 (Ebook)

First Printing Edition 2026

wisdom4mydaughtersbook@gmail.com

Dedication

For Morgan and Christina.

I love you more than any words could ever express.

Table of Contents

Preface

Dropping Morgan off at the University of Michigan in 2022, I hugged her goodbye and told her, "Remember everything I've taught you." When it came time to leave Christina at Michigan State in 2025, I realized I was repeating a ritual—leaving my youngest with the exact same hug and the exact same parting words. This moment with both of my girls is what led me to write this book. "Everything I've taught you" is a lot to remember!

Having lost my mother to Alzheimer's disease in 2020, I wish I had a compilation of all her wisdom written down somewhere. Since I don't, I decided to write down the wisdom I have gained in hopes that these bits of insight will help my children on their own journey. I could not have come this far without the love and experiential knowledge given to me by my mother. I want to share that gift with my daughters and I hope they will do the same for their own children.

This book is for my daughters, Morgan and Christina. I hope they will refer to it often. I want them to know I am writing it because I love them so much and truly want what is best for them always.

Life is a journey, a series of choices. Good choices lead to good outcomes. I have learned many truths about this journey, and I share these truths to help my girls and anyone else with their own life expedition.

These tidbits of wisdom come from a place of great love; a love I could never have experienced without becoming a mother. My intention is to advise my daughters from the most loving place in my heart and reveal the deepest truths I have discovered about what it means to live a good and meaningful life.

There are concepts I write about that I don't expect my daughters to fully understand until they are older. Several of the most important lessons I have learned are relatively new to me, having experienced exponential personal growth and enlightenment after I turned fifty. I do not expect my girls to thoroughly comprehend or apply later life lessons until they are around fifty themselves. We cannot understand certain things until it is time for us to understand them. When they're ready, I have left a little help here in these pages.

My wish for my precious daughters is that they live the very best lives they can. I hope this book is helpful in that pursuit.

Chapter One

Trust Your Gut.

My mother had a keen gut instinct. One winter night when I was eighteen years old, she specifically said, "I don't care if you go out tonight, but don't take your sister's car. I have a bad feeling about it." I told Mom I wouldn't take my sister's car, and she went to bed. An hour later, I left to hang out with my friends. Guess what car I drove? I figured everything would be fine, so I got into my sister's Geo Metro and drove to my friend's house.

I made it there without a scratch and proceeded to have a great time with my pals. It was well after midnight when I left. The roads were snowy with slick spots. I had almost made it home when I hit a patch of black ice. The car spun around a few times and ended up in a snow filled ditch. This was before cell phones. I was on my own. I tried to push the car out of the ditch, but it wouldn't budge. Luckily, a friend happened to drive by, saw me, and gave me a ride home.

The next morning, I woke up to my mother standing in my bedroom doorway. She said in a firm tone, "I don't care what happened or what you have to do. When I get home from work today your sister's car will be in the driveway."

Thank God for good friends. The same pals I had been hanging out with the night before saved me that day from the wrath of my mom. It took us all day to get the car out of that relentless ditch. We were finally able to get that little Geo back into the driveway about an hour before Mom arrived home.

I should have listened to my mother. I never doubted her instinct again.

Human beings are born with five senses: sight, smell, hearing, taste, and touch. However, there is another sense I encourage you to always trust. Some call it the sixth sense. Others call it intuition. I call it gut instinct. "Trust your gut," are the exact words I have used when advising you girls on this topic.

We periodically find ourselves in situations that feel scary or uneasy. Even when we cannot explain that uneasy feeling or fear, our gut instinct is the superpower that tells us something is wrong.

If your gut is telling you to get out of a place or situation because you are in danger, listen to it. I do not know how it works or why, but I know that your gut feelings will never steer you wrong. Trust your instincts. If you feel like you're in danger, you probably are. Confidently trust your superpower of intuition and learn to become in tune with it. If others doubt you, do not listen to them. Always trust your gut.

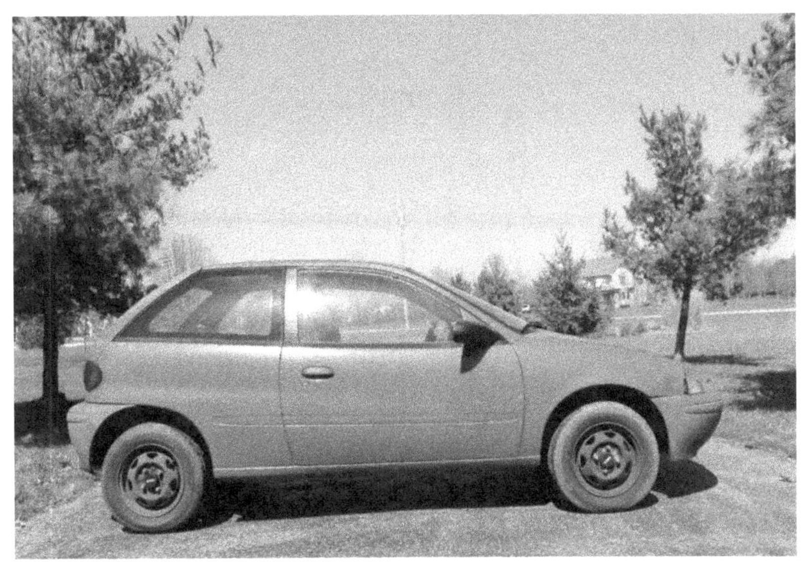

Pictured above: a Geo Metro just like my sister's.

Chapter Two

Exercise.

As an avid exerciser myself, I can testify to the many benefits that working out provides. I am stronger and more flexible because I exercise. I have maintained a healthy weight consistently throughout my years of fitness. My mind is clearer and more focused because of daily training. One of my favorite things about my workout is the "I did it!" feeling I get every time I finish. After twenty-eight years, I still get the rewarding feeling of accomplishment after every session. I admit I am addicted to exercise, and it is an addiction I am proud of.

Exercising regularly reduces the risk of heart disease and stroke. It decreases the risk of certain types of cancer and type two diabetes. Being physically fit improves blood pressure. It reduces high cholesterol and blood sugar levels. Obviously, working out strengthens our muscles and bones while increasing our flexibility and balance. These physical benefits help us to feel good every day.

The effect exercise has on our mental state of mind is helpful to our well-being. The phrase, "working out" is appropriate because while I'm working my body out, I am simultaneously working problems out in my mind. Physical training is a wonderful way to release stress. It makes us feel happier and decreases the risk of depression and dementia. Keeping fit enhances our cognitive functioning and memory.

Other advantages include a boost in energy and improved sleep. Our self-esteem goes up when we are fit, making us more likely to engage with other people and improving our social interactions. People who exercise have a prolonged life expectancy due to the physical and mental benefits it provides.

Many people do not feel motivated to work out. It can be difficult to get started. That is not an excuse not to exercise. Find a type of exercise you enjoy. Going to the gym is not for everyone, but a lot of people are very successful using a gym. Other options include running, finding routines you like on television or the internet, or playing a sport regularly. Take a Zumba or spin class. Try yoga. Dancing, walking, swimming, biking, hiking, or weight training are all good choices. There really is something out there for everyone.

Living a sedentary lifestyle is a prescription for a short and unhealthy life. Don't be lazy. Get up and get moving every day. This is one of the most important ingredients to a healthy and happy life. Find a way to enjoy your workout. Discipline yourself to exercise every day. You will be better in every way and you might even enjoy it.

Chapter Three

Cook at Home.

My mom taught me how to cook. We spent a lot of time together in the kitchen making all kinds of yummy food. When you eat my spaghetti, you're eating hers. Whenever I make beef-vegetable-barley soup, I feel a rush of loving memories of my momma. She always made it fun and included everyone at home in meal preparation. She loved simple foods and fancy foods alike – goulash was on the same level as stuffed beef tenderloin. Your grandmother was an excellent cook. I have tried to pass her kitchen know-how to you young ladies as best I can.

Eating well is not always convenient, but it is well worth the effort. It is tempting to grab a bite for lunch somewhere or go out to dinner instead of preparing our own meals. Financially speaking, the expense of eating at restaurants on a regular basis can add up quite a bit, pinching your pocketbook. The cost of eating out is high.

Our health pays an even bigger price. Eating out and eating processed foods has a negative impact on our bodies. Restaurants use a LOT of salt and other preservatives to make their food taste good. There are all kinds of nutritional deficiencies in processed foods including added salt, sugar, unhealthy fats, along with other harmful ingredients.

When we take time to prepare our own meals, our diet becomes markedly healthier. I have found joy in creating healthy meals for myself and my family. It feels good knowing I'm making food that will nourish us, keeping our bodies and minds in tip-top shape. I love to listen to Miles Davis, Chet Baker, or my Samba playlist while creating something delicious and ultra nutritious. It is even more enjoyable when the family cooks together. While it might feel like a chore at times, it can also be interesting and fun. I've enjoyed learning about food and how to prepare it in ways that enhance flavor and nutrition.

Vegetables are the superheroes of our diet. Find ways to make them delicious. Try different seasonings and cooking methods. Air frying is a great way to enhance the flavor of your veggies. Roasting vegetables is another tasty option. Salads are always good whether they are served warm or cold.

The overall effects of eating at home are tremendously beneficial. I am not saying we should never eat at restaurants. I love going out to eat! Just don't overdo it, certainly not every day. I recommend packing your lunch from home through the week instead of eating out. Plan your meals in such a way that dinnertime is a joy and not a burdensome chore. It might take practice, but it will pay off in big ways.

Grandma Marilyn's Beef Vegetable Barley Soup

I got this recipe from your grandma over the phone one day. My mother did not measure anything. She told me, "You'll know how much to put in." I have added clarifications here for you.

This is a hearty soup and the recipe serves 8-10. The soup keeps well and tastes delicious the next day and the day after. I love to make it on cold winter weekends. My mom loved this soup. I am reminded of her every time I make it. Enjoy!

Ingredients:

3 Large Beef Short Ribs

Celery (3-4 stalks)

Onion (1/2 large or 1 small)

1 Large Can Stewed Tomatoes

3 Cups Cooked Barley

Vegetables of Choice

- In a large pot, cover short ribs with water. (about 6 cups)
- Chop celery and onion and add to pot.
- Bring to a boil then turn down to low and cover.
- Cook until meat falls off the bone. (Grandma's recipe says at least 2 hours, but it has always taken me closer 4 hours to get the meat falling off the bone.)
- While the meat is simmering, cook the barley according to instructions on the package.

- Set cooked barley aside.
- Remove meat and cool completely.
- Add stewed tomatoes.
- Drain any excess water from the barley. Add strained barley to the pot.
- Add vegetables. I use corn, peas, green beans, and carrots. Frozen is as good as fresh and a lot easier. Start with ½ a bag of each vegetable. Add more if you prefer.
- Salt and pepper to taste.
- Continue to cook on low heat.
- Add completely cooled meat back to the pot.
- Serve when all the ingredients are evenly distributed.

Chapter Four

Get Enough Sleep.

When I was a young adult, I had FOMO (fear of missing out) if I went to bed too early. Now that I am older, I have FOMO about missing sleep if I stay up too late. Sleep has become the priority. I have reached a point in my life where sleep comes for me. Around 9:00PM every night, the Sandman comes and takes me to his Dream Realm. I fall asleep in seconds and enjoy quality slumber for most of each night. Usually, I get up to use the bathroom between 3:00-4:00AM. It is a struggle at times to get back to deep sleep afterward, but I do my best to rest and try to go back to sleep. I know I am better at everything if I've had a good night's sleep. That is probably true for you as well.

Americans sacrifice sleep more than almost any other thing. Our society is one that pressures us to go, go, go at all times. Get as much done as you possibly can every day! Accomplish! Produce! Succeed! There is ample pressure to perform and keep up. Something has got to give. Too often, it's sleep. I strongly advise against this common habit of our American society.

Our bodies heal themselves while we sleep. Sleep boosts our immune system, helping us to fight off infections and diseases. It regulates our hormones, reduces inflammation in the body, and supports tissue repair and regeneration.

Our minds are highly dependent on sleep to keep working properly. Sleep enhances cognitive function and is essential for memory, learning and problem solving. It improves our mood and reduces stress. Losing sleep increases the risk of mental health conditions such as depression and other mood disorders. We are more likely to make mistakes when we are sleep deprived. Getting enough sleep is essential to better decision making and good judgement.

People who get enough sleep enjoy a healthier life overall. They get sick less often, keep their weight under control, and are generally happier than those who sacrifice rest. I promise it is worth going to bed early and getting those seven to eight hours every night! I know how you ladies enjoy your slumber. Do not sacrifice sleep. Keep enjoying those zzzz's.

Chapter Five

Drink a Lot of Water.

When your Aunt Purt (Kathleen) and I were teenagers, we spent our summers at home together. Our mom worked at Spring Meadows Country Club as their Office Manager. One day, my sister was walking down the hallway from her bedroom into the dining room and she collapsed. I was frightened because nothing like that had ever happened. We were home alone and I didn't know what to do. I ran to my sister and tried to get her to "wake up". After a couple of minutes, I was relieved to see her open her eyes. We called our mom and she asked Aunt Purt a bunch of questions. Eventually, it was determined that my sister was dehydrated. We got her some water and toast, and she recovered.

There is no healthier drink option than water. The simple act of drinking water has a multitude of benefits on the human body. It is truly miraculous. The only thing that hydrates our bodies is water. Other drinks do not measure up and are even dehydrating. I know I have drilled this into your heads. I said this to you every day of your lives growing up, "Drink water, girls. It's lifesaving and life giving." Perhaps you remember the daily question before school: "Do you have your water bottle?"

Drinking water regulates our body temperature, lubricates our joints, and protects our tissues. It improves our cognitive function and boosts our mood. Moreover, it helps us to eliminate waste from our bodies.

It is wise to drink water while consuming alcohol. I recommend alternating - one cocktail then a glass of water. Better yet, a glass of water, a cocktail, then another glass of water. Staying hydrated while indulging in alcohol helps you avoid getting too drunk, which can be embarrassing and painful the day after.

Dehydration can cause damage to your kidneys and your brain. If left unchecked, it can even lead to death. To stay hydrated, we should be drinking half of our body weight of water in ounces every day. If you weigh one hundred pounds, you should drink fifty ounces of water per day. That is a lot of water! Take your water bottle with you everywhere you go. Make sure you fill it up often!

Chapter Six

Be Smart About Alcohol.

As I write this, you girls are in college. What a wonderful time of enlightenment and growth! You are stretching your wings and finding your way in the academic environment of university living. Your dad and I are so proud of you.

Along with academics, college offers other new and enjoyable experiences. This is the field where you learn how adults play. Often, that includes drinking alcohol.

Drinking can be fun. We loosen up when we indulge in a glass of wine or a cocktail. It makes us feel lighter, more talkative, and helps us to relax and laugh easier. This feeling of fun and ease is exactly what makes it risky. Humans have been consuming alcohol for centuries. For some, it is a self-prescribed medicine. For others, it is a way to relax and enjoy some recreation with friends. Either way, you must keep it in check.

Alcoholism is real. It runs in my family. My dad is a recovered alcoholic. His mother was also an alcoholic. I believe my dad's brother, David, was also an alcoholic. Studies have shown that alcoholism is genetic and certain people are more prone to it than others. It is a slippery slope, and I encourage you to discipline your use of alcohol.

Drinking too much destroys our lives. When alcohol becomes the primary focus, all relationships suffer. Decision making becomes warped and our priorities get all messed up. Our physical and mental health deteriorate along with our friendships and careers. I have seen the destructive power of alcoholism up close and personal. Many arguments between couples and friends erupt as a result of intoxication.

Hangovers are no fun, but excessive drinking can do a lot more harm than a headache in the morning. It can lead to unintended pregnancy, injuries, car accidents, legal troubles, and abusive behavior. There are people who get sentimental when they drink and there are others who get mean. Things get dangerous with a mean drunk. Keep yourself in check and watch the people around you. If you feel like things are getting out of hand, it's time to call it a night. Avoid getting involved in conflicts with drunk people. Be careful.

Your dad and I enjoy drinking socially, having an occasional beer after work or glass of wine while cooking dinner. We must monitor our own habits. There are times we take a step back and lay off drinking for a while. Dry January and Sober October are great times to take a month off and reset.

I'm sure you've heard the saying, "everything in moderation". When it comes to alcohol, please be sure you are setting realistic rules for yourself. Drink water between cocktails. (See Chapter Five - Drink a Lot of Water.) Set a limit.

Do not let drinking for fun become excessive. Do not use alcohol as an escape from your problems. It will only make things worse.

This is true of other substances as well, but alcohol is the easiest one to obtain so I use it as an example. Be conscientious about what you put in your body and your brain. You only get one of each. Don't abuse either. Choose wisely and take care of yourself.

Chapter Seven

Be a Clean Person.

Good personal hygiene is more important than you might think. Cleanliness helps prevent the spread of germs and illness, improving overall health. Being a clean person boosts your self-esteem and has a positive impact on your social life. We are more confident when we feel fresh and we are more approachable when we smell clean.

Let's face it - people are stinky. Shower or bathe daily. Use soap. Be thorough and wash every part of your body. Some parts need more attention – wash the areas where you sweat the most fully and completely. Get the hard-to-reach places and in between the crevices. Wear deodorant and refresh when necessary. Keep your body clean.

Occasionally, it's OK to skip the shower. If you're having a stay-at-home day or you don't feel good, it is fine to scurb out for a day. Don't take it too far. One day is fine. Two days is questionable. Three days is unacceptable. Make it a basic practice to shower every day.

Washing your clothes helps you stay clean. Clothing holds germs and odors that we emit throughout the day. Even if an article of clothing looks clean, it may not smell clean. Do your laundry!

Measure your detergent and use a booster like Oxi-Clean to keep your clothes bright and fresh. Use fabric softener so your clothes don't come out with static cling. Don't overload your washer or dryer. Be kind to your appliances. Fold your items nicely, preventing them from getting wrinkled. Put your clothes away. Don't leave them strewn about.

Wash your hands every time you use the restroom. This might seem elemental, but there are plenty of folks out there ignoring this basic principle. Whenever you are handling food, your hands should be freshly washed. After you've been wearing gloves or working outside, wash your hands. Use your common sense. Germs are tiny, that doesn't mean they aren't there. Remember to wash your hands!

Keeping a clean mouth is essential to the health of the rest of your body. Poor dental hygiene allows bacteria to spread from your mouth to the rest of your body. That can cause inflammation and infection. Believe me, you do not want to deal with tooth decay or other dental issues. Keep your dentist appointments to simple cleanings and regular check-ups. Avoid painful dental visits by taking good care of your oral hygiene every day. Brush and floss your teeth twice a day. Be thorough. Brush the back molars all the way around each tooth. Do not skip the flossing part. It helps you avoid bad breath, a socially undesirable condition. A white smile is more appealing than a dull, yellow or stained smile.

Be intentional and thoughtful about keeping your entire body clean and fresh every day.

Chapter Eight

Wear Sunscreen.

When I was still in elementary school, I fell asleep outside in the sun at the beach one day. I woke up with severe sunburn, especially on my face. It was painful and it took a long time to heal, peeling and itching every step of the way. This could have been prevented if I had applied sunscreen.

Seems like a no brainer, right? We Dugans are the whitest of the white people. When we go outside in the sun without sunscreen, we burn in minutes. This is not an exaggeration - it has happened to me enough times to know that I need to wear sunscreen each and every time I go out in the sun. So do you, my fair daughters.

There are folks out there who believe that wearing sunscreen is more dangerous than going out in the sun without it. Do not buy into this absurdity. Sunscreen protects you from getting skin cancer and helps you prevent your skin from aging prematurely. It reduces the risk of painful sunburns, sun sickness, and nausea.

Not all sunscreens are created equal, and some have harmful ingredients. Buy quality sunscreen. I recommend using sunscreen with zinc oxide or titanium dioxide. Neutrogena offers a few good options. Blue Lizard is another quality sunscreen, but it is a little more expensive.

Check the ingredients and look at customer reviews when you are choosing a sunscreen. Try to avoid products with oxybenzone or octinoxate methoxycinnamate, as these ingredients have been shown to disrupt the endocrine system. Do not settle for substandard sunscreens.

If you do get sunburned, treat it with aloe vera gel. Use cool compresses to relieve the heat. When your skin stops burning, use lotion to keep it moisturized through the healing process. Do not peel your skin. Allow it to peel off naturally. If you peel it, you may peel too much causing pain and possible infection. Be patient with your body to allow it to heal properly.

I know you ladies are disciplined about wearing sunscreen, but this is a topic that is so important I could not leave it out.

Keep a bottle of sunscreen in your car. This comes in handy in the spring and summer. Wear it on walks, at outdoor events and especially by the water or in high altitudes.

Your grandmother always told me the best sunscreen is make-up. I have found this to be true and even surprised my dermatologist with this sunscreen tip.

The first time I went to see my dermatologist he asked me if I had work done on my face. I laughed out loud and said, "No." He asked me why I don't have freckles on my face like I do on the rest of my body. I told him it's because I never go out in the sun without make-up on.

My momma was right. Wear face make-up when you go out in the sun. You'll thank yourself many years from now.

Chapter Nine

Be Proactive About Your Health.

During a visit to my doctor in 2022, I stepped on the scale. The nurse weighed me and measured my height. She said, "You're 5 feet 1 and ½ inches." My reply was, "No I'm not. I'm 5 feet 2 inches. I have been my whole life!"

I have Osteopenia which is a precursor for Osteoporosis. I would not have discovered I have this condition if I did not get a physical once a year. I learned about this by being proactive. I treat it with daily calcium and vitamin D3 supplements, preventing further damage to my bones. Thank goodness I found out with time to act! I have maintained my bone density for three years since discovering I have this condition. I am happy to report that I am maintaining a mighty 5 feet 1.8 inches. This reflects the 0.2 inches lost due to Osteopenia.

I know a few people who go to the doctor all the time. Personally, I do not like going to the doctor. I try to stick to my annual physical. This is a necessary yearly visit to make sure everything is working the way it should. If you take good care of yourself, hopefully you can just go one time each year. Annual health screenings are an important tool physicians use to monitor your health from year to year. Find a doctor you trust and partner with her to manage your health.

No one knows your body better than you. That includes doctors. Make sure you find a doctor who listens to you. Do not neglect that annual physical exam. Just do it.

Go to the dentist every six months to get your teeth cleaned. Do not wait until there is a problem in your mouth. It is easier and less painful to go to your semi-annual cleanings than having excruciating extractions, root canals or other unpleasant procedures. Plus, that beautiful smile is worth keeping fresh and clean.

As fair skinned people, I urge you to find a dermatologist and get a full body scan of your skin. Our sun is a powerful star and skin cancer is a real threat - especially to those of us who have pale skin. Get yourself checked once a year. Don't wait until there's a conspicuous spot somewhere on your body.

You might consider taking some supplements to boost your health. Our foods have been depleted of nutrients due to over farming. When farmers do not allow the land to rest once every seven years, the soil is depleted of essential vitamins and nutrients. This is why I take a multi-vitamin every day. I also take Vitamin C along with my Calcium and D3 supplements. There are other supplements in my daily routine, but I have not always taken them. I started taking Turmeric Curcumin to keep dementia at bay. Glucosamine helps me with joint pain as I age. I also take a B12 supplement that has reduced my back pain markedly.

Your father and I have had a few immunity infusions which offer a higher dose of vitamins and nutrients than we get from oral supplements. These infusions have helped both of us recover from or prevent common colds for the last couple of winters. We have both had great success and I highly recommend trying this method, especially during cold and flu season.

Don't wait until you're sick to go to the doctor. That is a reactive approach to your health. I do not mean to imply you should not seek medical care if you are sick. My point is you should get your annual physical as a proactive way to stay on top of your health. It is better to be proactive instead of waiting until you're sick or hurt and then being reactive. Be proactive about your health. I promise you will be better for it.

Chapter Ten

Keep a Clean House.

Your Grandma Marilyn worked full time and had to do all the housework on the weekends. Aunt Purt and I learned to help her when we were in our early years of elementary school. We had daily chores and weekend chores helping mom keep up with the house. That is how I developed a love for all things clean. Your Aunt Purt did not start out that way, but she eventually got there. I remember my sister's bedroom looking a lot like you girls' bedrooms throughout your adolescent years – definitely not my idea of "clean". It is ironically funny that your aunt became a professional cleaner later in her life. She is now one of the best homemakers I know.

Everyone who knows me knows I am a neat freak. My standards are ridiculously high. I do not expect you ladies or anyone else to hold to my outrageously high standards. Regardless, I encourage you to keep a clean home.

Every morning, I make my bed. It only takes a couple of minutes, and it makes a big difference in how the bedroom looks. I do one load of laundry per day. Mondays are dusting days. Every Tuesday morning, I clean my bathroom. I vacuum in the afternoon. The kitchen floor gets swept and mopped on Wednesdays. Thursday is grocery shopping day. Fridays are a catch-all for me because that is my day off.

The last thing most of us want to do after a hard day at the office is housework. Coming into an orderly space is much more conducive to de-stressing after a hectic day at work. We sleep better in a clean home due to this stress relief. Keeping the abode clean makes us more productive and puts us in a better mood.

I run my house like a job. I do a few different household chores each day. By doing a little bit every day, the house stays clean, and my mind remains clear. This way, I can spend my weekends and evenings focused on my family, not on cleaning.

Keeping a tidy house benefits everyone who lives there as well as anyone who visits. It is more comfortable to be in a clean area than it is to be in a dirty space. Obviously, keeping a clean home reduces allergens and germs that can make you sick. It improves the air quality and even reduces the occurrence of pests and insects.

When my house gets messy or cluttered, I feel like my mind is also in disarray. Mental clarity is easier to achieve when we are in a clear space free of unnecessary disorder.

I know this is more important to some people than it is to others, but I want to emphasize the physical and mental benefits of being a good home maker. If you don't want to clean or don't have time, I suggest hiring someone. It's a valuable service that's good for everyone in your household.

Don't neglect your home, take care of it. Keep it clean.

Chapter Eleven

Nurture Your Relationships.

Relationships are complicated. They can be wonderful to the point that we can hardly contain our joy and affection. Other times, well… relationships can be challenging and difficult. Either way, we need people. We need our family and we need our friends.

We are born into our families with no choice in the matter. Family relationships run deep and are generationally important. Our family ties can be weak or strong, depending on how we care for those ties.

The parent-child relationship is the most important for our development. This bond is the first emotional connection we experience and sets the stage for our emotional health. Often, grandparents play a critical role in the lives of their grandchildren. Your father was partially raised by his grandparents. Grandmas and grandpas are the best babysitters. Aunts and uncles can have an enormous impact on us. My own Aunt Le and Uncle Larry have been like parents to me. As you ladies know deep in your souls, the relationship you have with your sister is one of the closest bonds you will ever experience. It warms my heart to see how deeply you love each other. Don't ever let anything break that bond.

Respecting and honoring your parents is important and lays the foundation for future generations. Teach your children to be respectful of you and do not accept anything less as their mother. This is groundwork that will pay off in the future for everyone involved. Showing respect for parents is a lesson that will foster trust, empathy, and gratitude. Teaching children respect creates a harmonious home environment.

Honoring and respecting your children is equally critical to the parent-child relationship. Remember they are children, and they need guidance. We must respect and honor little ones as human beings with feelings, emotions and ideas of their own. This reciprocal relationship of honor and respect will bless both parents and children and ensure a lifelong love and reverence for one another.

There is an old saying about friends, "Some friends are for a reason. Some friends are for a season. And some friends are for a lifetime." Regardless of the type of friendship, they are all valuable and worthy of care. Spend time with your pals. Enjoy one another. Check in with each other. Friendships are important and should be attended to regularly.

There will be times when friends or family members disappoint you or let you down. While I do not advise anyone to remain in an abusive or destructive relationship, I do advise extending grace when necessary.

We are all flawed and every one of us makes mistakes. We need to give one another a second chance. Or a third. Maybe even a fourth. My point is people are worth forgiving and we are better off when we forgive. Do not throw people away when they make you angry or hurt your feelings. Work it out. Go through the awkward discomfort of having the hard conversations that lead to forgiveness and healing. Your relationships will be stronger as a result.

Chapter Twelve

Meditate.

It is hard to unplug and relax. We are inundated with a constant barrage of information on our phones. We're alerted to all the breaking news, super sales, upcoming events, natural disasters, and every political move our leaders make. These daily interruptions make it difficult to be present.

Our society tends to ignore the spirit and focus on the ego. The ego is a mechanism we need to survive in this judgmental and often cruel world. However, it is only a small part of what makes us who we are.

At the foundational core of our being, we find our true selves, our essence. When we shed the ego and get down to the actual soul of our being, we find we are designed for goodness and love. We are made to love one another, but our ego gets in the way. It is important to practice getting in touch with our true essence, putting our ego aside. We cannot get rid of our ego, but we can practice recognizing the difference between our ego and our essence.

The best method I have found to get in touch with my true self is meditation. Practicing meditation has been one of the most difficult habits for me to create because it requires a skill I am not great at, stillness.

I learned that meditating is important to my well-being and makes me a better person. It is not a waste of time or time spent doing nothing. It is an essential part of my spiritual life.

A couple years ago, I went through a difficult time that I named "menopause". I was in my early fifties and that seemed logical. My irritation level was high every day and I felt stressed out all the time. Nothing helped. I could not seem to break out of the dark cloud that was engulfing me. While I'll give hormonal changes their due credit, there was more contributing to my misery. I had lost touch with my true self and was becoming rigid, angry, unfulfilled and unhappy.

One of my closest friends, Dawn Russell, who also happens to be my boss and pastor, noticed I was suffering. She helped me get started on my meditation journey and take a close look at what was really going on with me. It was hard at first. But I kept at it in hopes that I could feel happy again, normal again, like myself again. As I continued to practice, I started to notice a change. I became calmer. Instead of feeling overwhelmed, I began to see things more clearly and realized I had been creating my own stress and sadness.

Dawn shared a book on the Enneagram with me. I learned about why I am the way I am, why I do the things I do, and what to do about it. Self-study is important, but incomplete without meditation. Only through my meditation practice, was I able to break away from my ego and rediscover my true essence.

I now meditate almost every day. Instead of waiting until I have checked everything off my list, I set time aside each day to meditate. Meditation has become more important than all those other things on my to-do list (See Chapter Ten - Keep a Clean House). I am happier, healthier and calmer. I am more in touch with my soul. Meditation is a gift we give ourselves to improve our spiritual health. That gift then extends to everyone else in our lives.

Don't let your ego get the best of you. Keep it in check by meditating regularly. You are more than the body you are in. We are beings of light made for goodness and love. Stay in touch with your soul.

Chapter Thirteen

Go to Church.

My Grandma (Pat) Morgan pressed it upon me as a young woman to "go to church". Back then, I was not at all interested in going to church. It seemed boring and I didn't like the idea of giving up my sleep-in Sunday mornings. At the time, I did not understand what my grandma was trying to do for me. I do now.

That was twenty-seven years ago. I have been a part of a church family for almost twenty-five years now and consider it to be one of the biggest blessings in my life. While I might not always agree with my fellow church members, these folks are my extended family. We gather every Sunday and worship our Lord and Savior. Jesus brings us together in ways we could never imagine possible.

The commonality we share as believers is the foundation of our care for one another. Jesus calls us to love and help each other. We are better equipped to do this when we worship and serve together in community. Our faith is a gift, and church is where we can engage with others to grow our faith and desire for God. It's not perfect - not by a long shot. However, it has had a positive effect on my marriage, my relationship with my children, with others, and my total outlook on life.

The church is like a family. Families can be dysfunctional. As church members, we are part of that fallible, dysfunctional family. Continually coming together and working together in Christ's service helps us to improve our relationships with others. It expands our understanding of one another. We can see the inherent goodness in each other despite our personal differences. This is what makes church important and helpful in our journey.

Being involved in a faith family helps us to grow in our understanding of God and spirituality. I have found this to be one of the most important aspects of life. Seeing how God works in each of us is enlightening. The support and love I receive from my church family is invaluable to me.

I have seen how meaningful the church becomes to us as we get older. Church is the main hub of interaction for many elderly people who may not have other opportunities for connection.

Even though it can be dysfunctional, people who go to church regularly experience less stress and anxiety. Church goers enjoy improved mental health, stronger marriages, and increased generosity. We also have a lower risk of many health issues and enjoy longer life spans than those who do not have a faith family.

In the words of your beloved Great Grandma Morgan, "go to church".

Chapter Fourteen

Spend Time in Nature.

We live in a world of busyness and stress. The constant pressure we feel is damaging. We need a path to serenity, and I have found that path to be nature. Spending time reconnecting with nature should be a daily priority.

My personal respite place is our boat. I call it my favorite room in the house. When I am on the boat, I am not distracted by anything. I am one with nature. My focus sets on the sounds, smells, and sights around me. There is abundant beauty to behold and I find myself in awe. The items on my checklist no longer feel as pressing and I can relax.

Our souls are restored by nature. The smell of the outside air, the sound of the birds chirping and the wind rustling the leaves on the trees summon us to reconnect with Mother Nature. We are part of nature, not separate from it. Acknowledge your part. Recognize that all of God's creation is connected. If one part suffers, all parts suffer.

The moment we step outdoors and surround ourselves with creation, our blood pressure goes down. Breathing fresh air reduces stress and anxiety. Spending time outside improves our mood, and we are more likely to be physically active outdoors. Our minds are nurtured by nature, reducing stress and improving our cognitive functions. We are less likely to develop mental illness when we connect with nature on a regular basis.

In a world where many people are ruled by their phones, it is crucial for us to remember to take time to detach from our technology and get back to our true selves. That true essence can only be found in the natural world and certainly cannot be found on a smart phone or computer.

Be sure to take time to get back in touch with nature. There are lots of options. Take a walk. Go to a park. Find a patch of grass to sit on. Go to the water. Hug a tree. Garden. Go to the beach. Your soul will be nourished by reconnecting with Mother Nature. I promise it's worth it.

Chapter Fifteen

Grow in Spirit.

There will be life events that will force spiritual growth in miraculous ways. Your father and I tried for over two years to conceive Morgan. The first time I miscarried, it resulted in an ectopic pregnancy and I had to have one of my fallopian tubes removed. That cut our chances of having a baby in half. I became laser focused on getting pregnant. Charting a calendar and taking my temperature daily, I would try to guess "just the right moment" to try and conceive with your dad. (Sorry if that's too much information, it is necessary for the story.) I took fertility drugs for six months. No baby. Then, another miscarriage. When the doctor told us the next step was in-vitro fertilization, we gave up. We couldn't afford the procedure. I thought I would never have children.

Guess what happened next! Oh baby!! That's when our Morgan came.

I had to surrender. I "gave it to God" as they say. Your dad and I did everything we could. Ultimately, it was not up to us. God's plan is a lot better than mine. When I stopped trying to control the situation, putting all my trust in God, that's when we successfully conceived. You girls are our little miracles! No event has ever grown my spirit like being your mom. Our souls are permanently connected. I felt it the day you were born and still feel it today.

Practicing meditation is an excellent way to grow your spiritual life. (See Chapter Twelve - Meditate.) However, it is not quite enough. Stay curious about your spirituality and find ways to satiate that curiosity.

I have enjoyed reading books that have piqued my interest and fed my desire to understand more about my spirituality. I started by reading about the Enneagram and learning about the nine personality types.

Discovering that my personality is a Type One helped me begin to understand my behavior. I learned that Type Ones are especially prone to anger and studied the psychology behind that anger. Becoming self-aware helped me to stop the anger from festering and turning to bitterness. I was able to face my constant need for perfection in a more healthy way, realizing my standards can be unreasonably high. This was enlightening and helpful in my effort to rediscover my true essence.

I still enjoy studying the Enneagram and find it to be extremely insightful regarding my own conduct as well as the behavior of others. My favorite book on the Enneagram is "The Wisdom of the Enneagram: The Complete Guide to Psychological and Spiritual Growth for the Nine Personality Types" by Don Richard Riso and Russ Hudson.

Another one of my favorite books is "Women Who Run with the Wolves: Myths and Stories of the Wild Woman Archetype" by Clarissa Pinkola Estes, Ph.D. The author uses stories and myths to discover deep truths about the female experience. She breaks down all the archetypes in each myth or story and explains the role each type plays in our lives. There is a historical truth in these legends that we all share in our human experience. I love the way she sheds light on the characters effect on us throughout our own life story. My favorite story in this book is called "The Red Shoes". It describes a girl who trades her authentic and instinctual life for a superficial, shallow existence that leads to self-destruction.

I just started reading "Radical Acceptance" by Tara Brach, a psychologist and Buddhist. I believe this is Tara's best work and I look forward to finishing the book. "Radical Acceptance" serves as a spiritual guide to help overcome feelings of unworthiness and shame. I love how open and honest the author is about her own experiences with these universal feelings.

If reading isn't your thing, try an audiobook or a podcast. I love listening to Tara Brach's podcasts. Her approach and style open my heart and mind in new ways. I am not always in the mood to sit down and read. Sometimes I'll listen to a podcast instead. Another favorite of mine is *Hidden Brain*, a podcast from NPR that reveals mysteries about the human mind. There are lots of ways and opportunities to grow in our spirituality. Find what works for you and continue to explore it.

Clearly, the Bible has been instrumental in my personal spiritual journey. I listen to scripture every morning while I eat my Cheerios. My Bible app tells me I've completed the entire Bible seven times now. I don't think I am a Biblical scholar, but I do tend to hold on to the words of Jesus Christ. The Old Testament points to Christ numerous times and I appreciate the lessons taught in the first half of the Bible. I especially love the book of Proverbs, written by King Solomon. Proverbs is a book of wisdom that provides excellent advice on how to live a good life.

I believe the Holy Bible was inspired by God Himself, but it was obviously written by men. Human beings have a way of skewing things to their own advantage. We are sinners after all.

The foundation of my faith is the message of Jesus Christ. Right now, I am studying the New Testament to focus solely on Christ's words. For me, the words written in red are the most important in the entire Bible. Jesus has never led me astray.

Your spiritual journey is intimate and personal. God comes to us in many different ways. Whatever spiritual path you take, study it. Read about it. Listen to it. Learn about your inner self. Remember you are mind, body, and *spirit*. Do not neglect the spiritual aspect of your life. You are beings of light. Shine brightly.

Chapter Sixteen

Beware of Social Media.

Instagram had my number. They knew exactly how to get my attention. My content was full of mostly politically related posts or anti-aging products and schemes. I would find myself heading down rabbit holes I never intended going down.

Anyone who knows me knows that the current political climate in the United States makes my blood boil. Instagram figured that out quickly and I started seeing more posts that were designed to make me mad. I am not a person who needs any fuel for my anger. I have quite enough anger regarding the political scene here in America to last the rest of my life. It is hard enough to maintain a healthy mental state as it is. Even when the posts I saw were in line with my thinking, they still elicited a negative response from me. This is deliberate on the part of Instagram and every other social media platform. They want you to keep scrolling. The content you see on these platforms is specifically chosen just for you based on your previous use.

As soon as I deleted my Instagram account, my irritation level went way down, and I stopped stressing about how to look younger too! Personally, I have found life considerably more peaceful since I stopped participating in social media. I understand there are good things that social media can provide. I also know how harmful it can be if you don't keep it in check.

I never created a Facebook account. I rarely look at my Linked In app. Tik-Tok has never been on my phone. There are many options to engage in social media, but I find all of them to be harmful. These platforms are studying your reactions and using your personalized algorithms to feed you content that you either love… or hate. This is why I stopped using social media. There is good media out there, but you must seek it out.

Now I spend time each day meditating, reading, and connecting with nature. This is better for me than any social media app could ever be. Instead of my blood pressure rising, I feel calmer, happier, grounded, and clear.

One of my favorite mentors, Tara Brach, says we live in a trance most of the time. We're focused on the future and constantly thinking about what we need to do next. It's like running in a race that we can never finish. Stop. Look around. Listen. Just be. The best gift you can give yourself is the present. Pay attention to what is happening around you - not what's on your phone. Take time to unplug every day. Be present with yourself and your physical surroundings. It sounds simple, but being present is a discipline that can be challenging due to the constant distractions we encounter every day. Sit outside. Listen to the song of nature. (See Chapter Fourteen - Spend Time in Nature.) Let your racing mind rest. Allow the flood of thoughts to pass by and be present. Put your phone down and find joy in the moment you are living.

Chapter Seventeen

Manage Your Money.

My mom was a financial wizard. I remember watching her as a little girl typing numbers into her adding machine. Her fingers hit those number buttons so fast I could hardly understand how she did it! Your grandmother had a fabulous relationship with numbers.

When I was fourteen years old, my mom began teaching me how to manage money. We would sit down at the kitchen table and go through the monthly bills. My mom allowed me to see her finances up close as she taught me how to prioritize the upcoming bills and plan for future expenses. I helped her balance her checkbook as she wrote the checks to be sent to the bill collectors. This was an eye-opening experience as a teenager to see how fast my mother's hard-earned money was spent. Your grandma taught me how to balance my checkbook and pay my bills.

Beware of credit cards. Using a credit card is fine if you pay it off immediately. In the words of your Papa Fisher, "If you don't have cash to pay for it, you can't afford it." Credit card companies charge high interest rates to make a profit. When you make purchases using a credit card, be sure you have the money to pay it off right away. Do not fool yourself into thinking you'll be able to pay it off later. That almost never happens. Unfortunately, I have experienced this in my own life more than once.

Credit card debt compounds as interest is charged each month. Before you know it, you are drowning in debt. It is extremely difficult to pay credit card debt off due to the monthly interest. Please heed my warning. Do not use credit cards unless you can immediately pay them off. I cannot stress this enough.

It is wise to keep a budget for yourself. Know what your monthly expenses are and budget your income. Give yourself a realistic allowance each month. Then, plan your expenses wisely.

I recommend putting some of your money in some type of savings account. If you can, invest your savings to increase it. Dad and I have an investment account through Edward Jones and have started accounts for both of you girls. Continue contributing to these accounts to save and make money. Use what you need to cover your bills and monthly expenses. Give a designated amount to whatever charity you choose or the church you decide on.

Money is necessary, but it can make life stressful. Manage it correctly and do not live beyond your means. Be realistic about what you need and what you can afford. Give some away and make sure to save some for a rainy day.

Chapter Eighteen

Love Your Job.

I am happy both of you young ladies are achieving your academic goals. You are smart, energetic, creative people and you are on the right track to success. When you finish college, it will be time to begin your careers.

There are plenty of folks who hate their job. This is unfortunate because we spend quite a bit of our lives working. Life is too short to spend doing a job that is unfulfilling or miserable. I suggest finding a career that holds your interest and curiosity. Work in a field you enjoy. They call it work for a reason, but it does not have to be dreadful.

My first career was in insurance. I answered a "help wanted" ad in the newspaper when I lived in Novi. The job opening was for a clerk in an insurance agency. I worked as a clerk in that office for two weeks before my new boss told me he would pay for me to get my agent's license. I obtained my license less than a month later. Immediately, my income went up considerably. The new title of "insurance agent" made me feel important and boosted my confidence.

The insurance industry was good to me for a long time. I worked for Farmers Insurance Company for the first two years and then moved up to a larger independent agency that represented many insurance carriers.

Having started in personal property and casualty insurance, I soon moved up to servicing commercial clients. Moving up the ladder felt good, but the job got increasingly stressful. My workload never got smaller, it got bigger every day. The pressure was more than I could take.

After a few weeks of coming home in tears every day, your dad said to me, "I just want my happy wife back." He supported me in my decision to leave the industry. This was a scary time for me because a lot of my identity was wrapped up in my career.

Your Aunt Purt and I started a cleaning company together. We called it Two Sisters Housekeeping. The business got off to a slow start, but we eventually had a regular clientele and were making enough to get by. We enjoyed working together and my job, although not as prestigious, was no longer a source of stress.

It was during the time I was working with your Aunt Purt that I got pregnant with Morgan. I worked until my seventh month of pregnancy. Once Morgan came into the world, I stopped working to become a stay-at-home mother. Thankfully, I stayed home with you girls until Christina started Kindergarten.

Instead of going back to the world of insurance, I landed an awesome job as a teacher at a little preschool in Davisburg. What an absolute delight it was to work with all those adorable children! I loved working with the toddlers.

Working as a preschool teacher was not the most lucrative job, but it was rewarding in many ways. I made a small difference in the lives of the children I taught. That was more fulfilling than anything I ever did in the insurance industry.

While I was still teaching preschool, the opportunity to work at the church fell into my lap. Feeling called to this position; I jumped at the chance I had been given. I was hired by Linden Presbyterian Church in May of 2015. Working in the church has been the most fulfilling and rewarding job I have ever had. Helping people in our community and serving the church has blessed me immeasurably. I have never been happier at work than I am now. I do not make big bucks, but I am rich in every way that truly matters. My work is important to our community, and I feel great about the work I get to do.

The best advice I can offer you girls about work is to find something you love to do and then figure out how to make money doing it. I know you are both on track to work in your desired field and I could not be prouder of you. Keep up the good work!

If you find yourself feeling unfulfilled or unhappy in your work life, remember you have options. You can change careers. Do not feel like you must keep working at a job that makes you miserable. Don't quit your job until you have another one. There are a lot of jobs out there. You can do whatever you want. Do not hate your job. Love what you do for a living.

Chapter Nineteen

Don't Worship Money.

For many years, I thought I wanted financial wealth. Often, I silently lamented that I couldn't afford new clothes, expensive beauty products I thought I needed, or vacations to tropical destinations. My biggest financial woe was our house. I wanted new floors in our home, and it was always just out of reach because there were many other things that took precedence. My least favorite chore was sweeping and mopping that kitchen floor because it was in disrepair and I wanted new floors badly! I would get angry and feel a sense of unfairness.

Well, as we all know, life isn't fair. As the Grandpa states in *The Princess Bride,* "Who said life is fair? Where is that written?"

Money is necessary. We need it to survive. However, the societal focus on money and power has been destructive to our families and our nation. Seeing the negative effect money has on people makes me reconsider my old desire for wealth.

When I think about what makes me happy and fulfilled, money is never the first thing that comes to mind. It is my family that is the most valuable to me. My friendships come in a close second. The relationships we have in this life are what matter most.

I have observed that when people gain wealth, they often lose humility and forget what it's like to struggle. They become prideful and start to think of themselves above others. The desire for more money is never satiated. This is an ego-driven mentality that suffocates the soul and puts barriers between the rich and the poor. It serves no good purpose and hurts everyone.

It would be unfair of me to throw every wealthy person under the bus. There are affluent people out there doing enormously good things with their fortune. MacKenzie Scott has donated over $26 billion focused on education and economic equity.

Charles Stewart Mott is another example. Mott is the founder of the Charles Stewart Mott Foundation. The original purpose of the foundation was to improve the community of Flint, MI. Now, the foundation continues to focus on the Flint area including funding programs for youth, the environment, and civil society.

Conversely, a great number of people who gain financial wealth do not give their money away to make the world a better place. Many just keep getting richer and do not do anything to help anyone else. To me, this is morally and ethically wrong on every level.

Perhaps there is a psychological shift that happens when people get ultra rich. It is like they forget there are people out there who are hungry, without shelter, needing medical treatment, and trying to feed their families.

This chosen amnesia is prevalent in America today and is intensifying as the chasm between the wealthy and the poor continues to get bigger.

Remember where you come from. Think about the needs of others. Remember there are a lot more people in the middle class and among the poor than there are billionaires. We should all be taking care of each other, not hoarding all the riches for ourselves. Besides, who on Earth needs that much money in the first place? I have heard that the wealthiest people in the world are also the most unhappy. Their friendships are based on what people can get from their rich buddy, not real connections. Sounds kind of awful, doesn't it?

One of my favorite quotes is from our next-door neighbor, Brian. He said, "Money screws people up. I'm glad I don't have any!" Well said, Brian, well said indeed.

If I had unlimited wealth, I would donate to organizations that address climate change and mental illness. I would probably buy a new car too. I'm not perfect. Still, I hope I would give most of it to non-profits and groups that benefit people and the world. I think it is OK to treat yourself for your successes, but balance that out by donating to worthy causes.

If you find yourself making more money than you need, find a way to make the world a better place. Help others who have nothing. Do the right thing and don't get prideful. We don't get to take anything with us when our time comes to meet our maker. You will bless others and be blessed yourself when you show generosity instead of greed.

Chapter Twenty

Don't Compare Yourself with Others.

Sheryl Crow sums this idea up beautifully in her song, "Soak Up the Sun", saying, "It's not having what you want. It's wanting what you've got."

As I go along on my own journey, I find that comparing my situation to others is never a good idea. It is a natural tendency for human beings to compare themselves with other people, but this is harmful.

Things are not always as they appear. I might think someone has a better lot in life than me, but I'm not seeing the whole picture. Everyone has problems and no one's life is perfect. The folks I compare myself to may also compare themselves to me. They might think I have something better than they have. What a vicious cycle of unnecessary envy! We all get a different hand in this game of life. Some people have a big, beautiful house. Other people have a warm, loving family. Yet others get next to nothing! We can only play the cards we are dealt.

I have an awesome family and many close friends. I would not exchange that for all the money in the world. Still, I know I have compared my home, car, clothes, education, and job to others who I have viewed as having it "better" than me. Making this unrealistic comparison is not good for anyone. Ultimately, it makes us feel inadequate.

You are not inadequate. You are enough and you have enough. Be grateful for what you have been blessed with in your life. Do not be fooled into thinking your life would be better if it resembled someone else's.

Life is what you make it. Your unique and wonderful existence is like no other. Gratitude is a better option than jealousy. Don't waste your time trying to "have what you want". Instead, "want what you've got." You've got enough.

Chapter Twenty-One

Be Authentic.

When I was in elementary school, every year I would meet my new teacher and they would say, "You're Kathy's sister, aren't you?" All the teachers loved my sister. All our family members and friends did too. Being compared to my older sister throughout my childhood often made me feel like I should be more like her. I tried for many years to be like your Aunt Purt. What I discovered is this is impossible. I am not my sister. I am Melissa. Aunt Purt and I share our parents and upbringing and many other things, but we are very different people.

It took me a long time to feel comfortable in my own skin. If I am not my sister, who am I? Once I stopped trying to be someone else, I had to figure out who Melissa is. This created conflicts in me because it felt like I was going to disappoint the folks who seemed to think I should be like your Aunt Purt. Realizing I would never be anyone other than myself forced me to take that chance. It turned out my family and friends liked and accepted me for who I am and I began to feel more at ease. I began accepting Melissa for who she is.

For the majority of my adolescent life, people pointed out my fair skin as if it is some kind of detriment. "Get a tan," is a comment I've heard lots of times. None of us gets to choose the color of our skin.

This constant feeling of inadequacy due to my fair skin was a bit tormenting for me, especially in my late teens and early adulthood. What did I do about it? I started tanning at a tanning salon. I was able to achieve a decent tan, but at what cost? We all know tanning is bad for us. The pressure I felt to be tan, like everyone else, was enough for me to take the risk. Looking back on it now, I wish I felt more confident in my fair skin. The older I get, the more I prefer my natural pale skin than a forced tan.

I am not my sister. My natural skin color is porcelain white. My name is Melissa Dugan and I have come to love Melissa just as she is. It has taken me almost my whole life to truly accept myself for who I am.

When we feel like we don't fit in, we are tempted to act like someone else to be accepted into a social group. There are times other people in your life will tell you you're doing something wrong or you should do things differently. Do not feel trapped by people wanting you to be something you are not. Remember, there are lots of ways. (See Chapter Thirty-One - Keep an Open Mind.) We can only be ourselves. Trying to imitate others or act in ways that are contrary to our true selves is exhausting and, frankly, dishonest. Be true to yourself for your own benefit as well as the people in your life.

When we are free to be our true selves, we offer that freedom to others we come into contact with. Authentic people are drawn to others who are genuine. There is something attractive about quirkiness and honesty that makes people curious.

Unfortunately, authenticity is a rare quality. When we interact with those who are genuine, we feel a sense of trust and reverence for them. In this age of productivity and performance, we often see people wearing a variety of masks to feel accepted and valued. Many are afraid to show the world who they really are.

Always be true to yourself. You are beautiful, smart, kind, talented, interesting and unique women who have a lot to offer this world. Do not ever feel that you need to be something or someone you are not. God created you as the amazing people you are. There is no one else like you. Never compromise your authenticity. Be yourself. Be authentic.

Chapter Twenty-Two

Have Fun.

There never seems to be a shortage of things we have to do. Why do we work so hard? Clearly, we have to pay our bills and earn money to buy food, clothing, and take care of our other basic needs. When all the necessities are taken care of, I suggest taking time to have fun. In fact, I recommend taking as much time as you can for enjoyment.

I live for fun. Anticipating spending time with friends and family helps me get through the work week. What is the good of living without fun? Life is short. We should enjoy it as frequently as possible.

My mom was a great example of how to make mundane things fun. She taught me to jam out to good tunes and dance while cleaning the house. I still rock out to Dave Matthews Band, Van Halen, or Kenny Chesney when I do my chores. It was my mom who showed me and my sister that doing the dishes together could be a time filled with laughter and fun. When we spend time with the people we love, it does not matter what we're doing. Everything is more enjoyable when we do it together.

Fun is the reward we get from our hard work. There is nothing like meeting up with friends on a Friday evening after the work week comes to an end. It is delightful to enjoy a meal and have a few laughs together.

Play games. Start a project. Do a puzzle together or work on a craft. This is what makes the weekends awesome. It is our time to focus on family, friends and fun. We look forward to this fun break every week. It helps us push through our work and to-do list with a more positive attitude and a sense of hope. Without fun, life would be mundane. What would we look forward to?

Our busyness can get in the way of our fun. Prioritize fun in your life. I do not mean you should neglect your other obligations but be sure to allow for fun time. It is critically important for your well-being.

Sprinkle a little fun in everything you do. Work is work, but it doesn't have to be miserable. Go into things with a positive attitude and try to enjoy whatever you're doing. One way to make your job more fun is to make friends at work. My boss, Dawn, is one of my best friends. Our friendship makes my work fun. In the words of my favorite songwriter, Dave Matthews, "Turns out it's not where, but who you're with that really matters". Surround yourself with good people and be a positive force. Be deliberate about enjoying yourself. Have fun on purpose.

Chapter Twenty-Three

Manage Stress.

Before I met your father, my life was full of tension. I wasn't taking very good care of myself. My career was important to me, but the job was one of unrelenting high-pressure. My methods of dealing with it were smoking, drinking, staying out too late and eating unhealthy, comfort foods. What a recipe for disaster! I was not in good health. My blood pressure was high, and I started to gain weight. I felt sick all the time because my lungs were struggling. This was a turning point in my life. I realized if I did not change my ways, my life was not going to be the one I had always dreamed of.

I started working out when I was twenty-five. That was the first step toward a healthier lifestyle. Next, I quit smoking. It felt good to breathe freely again and I stopped getting sick. My drinking habit diminished significantly after I met your dad. As I got healthier, I got happier.

It was when I was trying to get pregnant that I changed my eating habits. The stress of not conceiving at first worked against me, creating more anxiety. Fearing I would never be able to have children compounded the pressure. The doctors told me I could not have children unless we did in vitro fertilization.

After several miscarriages, I began to wonder if my diet was contributing to my infertility. I learned about nutrition and started eating differently. I quit my high-pressure job and changed careers. Letting go of the need to control the situation was the turning point that led to acceptance. When I finally surrendered, I got pregnant with Morgan. I feel certain these lifestyle changes made it possible for me to have you girls.

Stress triggers your body's fight or flight response, leading to chronic physical issues like heart disease, high blood pressure and digestive problems. It is linked to memory loss, anxiety, depression and insomnia. Cortisol, the stress hormone, is released by our adrenal glands in response to stress. This hormone wreaks havoc in our bodies. It increases blood sugar levels and suppresses the immune system. Cortisol increases heart rate and blood pressure. The stress hormone promotes fat storage, weakens our bones, and disrupts our sleep. Whew! That is a lot of damage!

All these physical issues create more stress. Compound stress is like compound interest on a credit card. Nobody wants it.

Due to the catastrophic effects of stress, it is important to develop and maintain practices that help us reduce tension. There are a lot of options, and I recommend doing more than one thing to maintain your calm. I have touched on several of these practices already, but they are worth repeating.

Exercise. This is the best way I have found to blow off steam. (See Chapter Two - Exercise.) Pushing your body to its limits can really help relieve stress and frustration. Exercise regularly to keep stress at bay.

Meditate. You <u>can</u> control your thoughts. (See Chapter Twelve - Meditate.) Meditation is a practice that has helped me slow down my racing mind and focus on the present moment. It has been a wonderful tool to calm down and reset.

Get enough sleep. Remember our bodies heal while we sleep (see Chapter Four - Get Enough Sleep.) It is crucial in managing stress levels. We are more stressed out when we're tired.

I am a super healthy and happy person now. Taking care of myself feels good and the results benefit me and everyone else in my life. The actions we take to manage stress benefit us in every way. I implore you ladies to take this seriously and monitor your stress levels. Find methods of managing stress that work for you.

Chapter Twenty-Four

Keep Your Mind Sharp.

I love to play solitaire. It is a great way to keep my brain engaged. Moreover, it reminds me of my mother. She played all the time and taught me every game she knew. Whenever I play, I feel like she is sitting at the counter with me playing her own game while I play mine. This is how I feel close to my mom now that she is gone. I do not go to the cemetery, I play solitaire.

Our minds need exercise just like our bodies. Keeping your mental acuity sharp gets more challenging as you age. It's important to maintain your brain power by taking part in activities that keep your brain engaged.

There is an app called Lumosity that I highly recommend. It offers a wide variety of games to play that keep your mental abilities keen. There are sorting games, word and letter games, color coding games, and memory activities.

Another way to stay sharp is to play with words. I have always enjoyed the art of writing and using words creatively. As you know, I am a team leader on Wordscapes. I started playing Wordscapes on my phone when I used to pick you girls up from school. It was a great way to spend the time waiting in the parking lot for you to be excused for the day.

I've been playing for such a long time, my brilliance level is up to 1,086,990! Crossword puzzles and word finds are fun too. The more challenging, the better.

Numbers aren't always my niche, but I still try to do my own math instead of resorting to a calculator. Sudoku is a fun number game along with card games, Uno, and dice. Playing Yahtzee and Greed are some of my favorite games to play with family and friends.

Reading is one of the best ways to maintain a healthy brain. Try a variety of reading material. Read fiction for fun and read non-fiction books that will help you grow in your journey. Writing is another excellent way to keep your brain working at its best. Keep a journal. Write letters. Give creative writing a shot. Who knows? Maybe one day you will write a book!

My very favorite ways to stay sharp involve other people. Play games with your family and friends. Euchre is a Michigan favorite that challenges our strategic and mathematic skills. Dugans love dice games! Dominoes is a nice alternative to dice. Make plans to have a new adventure. Prepare a meal together. Try a recipe you've never made before. Do new things and go to new places. It's fun and keeps life interesting.

One of the best things you can do for your mind is to go outside. (See Chapter Fourteen - Spend time in Nature.) Spending time outside realigns our minds and helps us reconnect to our earth and the rest of creation. This simple act inspires new ideas and helps us resolve problems.

Make a daily habit of sharpening your mind. This should be fun, yet a little challenging. Forming this daily practice will pay off in big ways, especially as you enter your golden years.

Chapter Twenty-Five

Be Humble, Yet Confident.

Early in my insurance career, I found myself humbled. Starting a new job at a big agency, I felt like I was awesome. There was a pile of paperwork in the corner of my new office. I did not pay attention to it because nobody had said anything to me about it. When I finally looked at the stack of papers, I realized it was full of work I should have taken care of. Due to my neglect, I missed important things that were time sensitive. My new boss had to call me out on it and I was embarrassed. I felt small. I no longer felt like I was awesome. I was humbled. Just like every person, I made a mistake.

There is nothing wrong with confidence. If we are good at something, we can feel confident about it. When we work hard at learning and/or mastering a skill, we have every reason to feel secure in our abilities.

Do not forget you are human. Human beings make mistakes. I make mistakes every day. When you notice other people slipping up, extend grace. Keep in mind that we all slip up from time to time. You ladies are extraordinary. You are still fallible people. Do not allow your head to get prideful or swollen. No one likes a pompous or prideful show-off. Don't be arrogant. Be humble.

Humility is a desirable quality, and it is always a good idea to keep ourselves in check. While I don't want either of you ladies to get a big head or think too highly of yourselves, I also want you to be confident in the remarkable young women you are. It is important for us to recognize our value and strengths while remaining humble.

Our confidence can be squashed by others. When people feel inferior, they may try to put you down. They may try to make you feel inferior about yourself or your abilities. Insecurity can make people act in destructive ways toward others. Do not let jealous or envious people bring you down. Often, it is their personal self-doubt driving their actions. We should pray for those who fall into this destructive behavior. Realize it is their issue, not yours. We must maintain a thick skin for our own self-preservation. Emotionally driven comments from insecure, jealous individuals should be considered with skepticism. Always remember, hurt people hurt others.

Hold your head high, confidently knowing you are the best you can be. Don't forget the path that led you to where you are now. Hold on to your humility while standing tall in the self-assurance you have earned.

Chapter Twenty-Six

Be Compassionate.

I am blessed to be employed by a church whose mission is to help people in our community. The fulfillment I feel when I help people who are hungry or people who need help paying their rent is immeasurable. People need to tell their stories. When I take the time to listen to them with compassion, they are appreciative. Our clients are blessed by our food pantry and the financial assistance we provide. The gratitude they show us is genuine and heartfelt. We develop relationships with these clients, creating real community. No salary amount could ever compare to the fulfillment helping people provides.

Our culture is selfish. People in the United States tend to rely solely on themselves and their own resources. It feels like everyone is looking out for number one. Many are perfectly capable of taking care of themselves and their families without assistance. There are others who simply do not have the means to be independent. We need to have compassion for those who are less fortunate and do what we can to help them. (See Chapter Twenty-Seven - Serve.)

When we succeed in life, it is easy to get prideful. It is important to remember that none of us gets to our desired outcome by ourselves.

Our parents help us get our start in this world. We have teachers, colleagues, friends, and others who help us along the way. Let's not forget our Lord and Maker, who gave us life in the first place. No one has a right to be boastful. We are all dependent on someone or something for our growth and success.

There are many people suffering in the world. Families living in substandard conditions due to poverty need help. When impoverished families are stricken with illness, it is devastating to them. Medical bills and the need for medicine take priority over buying food, leaving family members hungry. Many of the poorest people in our communities are suffering from mental illness, making it nearly impossible for them to hold a job. People who are abused or neglected need help getting away from their abusers. It is difficult to start over, especially when you have nothing.

The challenges of living in poverty compound on themselves, often resulting in homelessness. Consider how difficult it must be for someone who is homeless to get a job. They cannot put an address on their application. Often, our homeless brothers and sisters do not smell good because they do not have means to properly take care of their personal hygiene. They do not have a place to take a shower or put a fresh change of clothes on for any kind of interview.

These patterns of living are passed down from generation to generation. If you are born into homelessness, the hope of a brighter future is bleak. For these folks, the only way out of homelessness is for someone to intervene and offer help.

If you encounter someone who is struggling, have compassion for them. Think about what it would be like to be in their situation. Don't think of yourself as better than those who are not as successful as you. None of us has control over the circumstances we are born into.

Pray for the poor. Pray for the sick. Pray for the elderly. Pray for the homeless. Even if you've never met them, pray for them. These are the outcasts in society, and they have the most need. Have compassion on these brothers and sisters of ours. We are all in this together and we need to help each other in this world. Remember, what comes around goes around. Be compassionate to those in need.

Chapter Twenty-Seven

Serve.

An amazing thing happens when we help people. Our perceptions of our own problems change when we assist others in need. While we bless people by serving them, they bless us too. This is the kind of connection our world desperately needs. The state of our nation is one of division right now. Helping one another and serving together is the path back to connection and reconciliation.

When we're in the thick of life, working and raising kids, it feels like there is no time left for anything else. Do not be fooled. We can always find time to serve in a small way.

Serving doesn't have to be a long or recurring time commitment. Find something you can do to help others. Volunteer at a local food bank, helping sort and put food on the shelves. Take clothes to a children's closet. Serve dinner to the homeless at a shelter or sit down with them to enjoy a meal together. Many elderly people in nursing homes do not have any visitors and don't receive any greetings from the outside world. Take cards to folks in a nursing home or make time to visit. Help an elderly neighbor with their yardwork or groceries. Stop to check in on them. There are infinite ways to get involved.

Volunteering improves our mood because it feels good to help other people. Serving others reduces our stress levels, again putting our own life in proper perspective. It enhances our self-esteem and reduces depression and anxiety. Volunteering contributes to more meaningful relationships, building stronger communities and reducing feelings of isolation and loneliness. We are happier when we serve.

Your dad and I have had many wonderful experiences serving our community. We have enjoyed heading up to the Food Bank of Eastern Michigan with other folks from church and working together to help however we could. One of our favorite organizations to volunteer for is Carriage Town Ministries. Carriage Town offers food and shelter to homeless people while giving job training and helping folks get their lives back on track. We have served dinner, scrubbed floors, and cleaned their sanctuary. It feels good, and we always have fun.

As you ladies know, your father and I have been serving in our church praise band for over twenty years. We love serving in this way with our long-time friend and drummer, Jarrod. All of us are passionate about music and our friendship has grown deeper over the years of working and playing together. We have been blessed to have several other talented musicians join us over the years. Playing and singing music in praise of our Lord has blessed us tremendously.

Being a part of our worship services ensures we are at church every Sunday, which is extremely helpful in our spiritual journey. It would be easier to stay home and sleep in if we were not committed to serve in this way. This commitment has helped your dad and I stay on track in our Christian faith. We have enjoyed strengthening relationships with our brothers and sisters in the church by regularly being present.

Last spring, your dad and I volunteered at the Fenton Pride Festival. We feel like the LGBTQ+ community has been treated unfairly by many people in government, schools, and even churches. This was an excellent opportunity to help a group of people who have been targeted by others as being "bad" or "unacceptable". We are all children of God and should all be treated with dignity and respect. It felt great to help out at that event and we met several lovely people in the process.

A lot of the volunteering we do for the Chamber of Commerce is just plain fun. We love to be out in the community talking to people and helping others. Your dad's involvement in the Chamber has been a blessing in that we have met many friends and had a lot of fun serving with others who participate in community events. I have enjoyed serving at the Taste of Fenton, the ServePro Send Off Party, and the Fenton Farmer's Market. All these events focus on bringing people together to form a close-knit community.

When we break out of our own little world and serve those around us, everyone wins. It's an opportunity you don't want to miss. There are limitless opportunities to help others. Find what works for you and serve.

Chapter Twenty-Eight

Be a Good Communicator.

There is only one way to let someone know what you're thinking or feeling. You must tell them. It can feel awkward, especially when the reason for your trouble is something the other person said or did. While it might seem easier to just let it go or ignore the issue, it will fester if you don't deal with it. Your relationship will be stronger if you just tell the person what is going on and explain why you feel whatever you're feeling. Do not assume they know. They don't and they can't. Speak up. Work through it. Be clear without being hurtful.

Many years ago, I had a conversation with my best friend, Beth. I was telling her how angry I was at my boyfriend at the time and how "he should just know" what was wrong with me. She interjected, "but he doesn't". This caught me off guard because I was used to Beth taking my side. She said, "how can he know you're upset if you don't tell him?"

Since that day way back in high school, I have seen many people fall into the same, "he should just know" trap. When we are in an intimate relationship, whether it be romantic or platonic, we sometimes assume the other person in the relationship automatically knows what we are thinking or feeling. Do not make assumptions about what other people are thinking. Just because someone knows us well, doesn't mean that person knows exactly what's going on with us.

Clear, honest communication is critical for any and every healthy relationship. No one can read your mind; even our closest friends are not mind readers. For people to know what we're experiencing, we must verbalize it. Speak it out loud.

If you feel like someone you're close to is upset with you and they aren't talking, say, "Are we OK? Have I done something to upset you?" There are ways to go about this that don't feel like confrontation. I recommend starting the conversation with an "I love you". Hold the other person's hand. It's hard to be angry at someone who just said they love you and is holding your hand. Always put love first, then start talking. Try to avoid coming from a place of anger. Remember the person you are in relationship with is not trying to hurt or offend you. We're all human beings and we make mistakes all the time. Extend grace when it's appropriate, but don't be doormat. Speak up for yourself when it's necessary.

It can be helpful to use the words, "I feel" when we are working problems out with others. "I feel like ____ when ____ happens." Avoid using extreme words like always and never.

Listen when that is what needs to be done. Being a good listener is a critical ingredient in healthy communication. There will be times when all that is required is listening. Use words when necessary. When it's time to listen, be present and focused on what is being said to you.

Communication is a two-way street. It requires expressing yourself and listening to others. Be honest about your feelings. Be patient and understanding with others as you listen to them. This will result in healthy relationships that last a long time.

Chapter Twenty-Nine

Choose Your Friends Wisely.

When you girls were little, I would tell you, "Not everyone is good." This, unfortunately, is a truth we must understand. There are a lot of wonderful people in this world, and there are also people who would hurt anyone to get ahead. Sometimes, it's obvious. Other times, we can be deceived by people pretending to be our friend when they actually have ill motives. This is especially true when someone is jealous of you. Jealousy is one of the most destructive motivators.

We Dugans are a social bunch. Family and friends mean the world to us, and we cherish the time we spend together. Life is richer and more pleasurable with people to share it with. Occasionally, we get burned by someone we think is our friend.

Your Papa Dugan says it this way: "Sometimes you gotta cut out the dead wood." If the relationship is damaging you, it's time to cut out the dead wood. Be sure not to over-trim, remembering to extend grace when it is appropriate (see Chapter Eleven - Nurture Your Relationships.)

If you find yourself in a friendship that makes you feel bad or inadequate, take time to investigate what is going on. What is causing that feeling? Is the person in question a good friend? Are they going through something they need help with? Do they lift you up and support you, or do they put you down? Is the relationship reciprocal, or does it feel one sided? If you're doing all the work in the friendship, that is not a healthy relationship.

There have been times I thought I was making a good friend and later discovered the friendship was not what I had hoped for. Early in our church life, I tried to strike up a friendship with a lady who was coming to church at that time. She was always nice to me, but I started feeling a bit like a lost puppy at her heels. I wanted to be her friend, but she was not reciprocating my efforts to become closer. Feeling slightly foolish and embarrassed, I stopped trying to earn her friendship. Relationships require reciprocal involvement. She was not ready or willing to reciprocate. I let her go. Reciprocal does not necessarily mean 50%-50%. It does mean consistent effort is being put into the relationship by both parties.

Right around the time I met your dad, a friend disappointed me in a more hurtful way. This young woman had a crush on your father. Your dad had a crush on me. She lied about me to other friends of mine. That girl wanted your dad, and I was in her way. It became clear that her friendship with me was not genuine. She was dead wood that needed to be cut out.

My lifelong friend, Beth, is and has always been the very best friend I have ever had. She has loved me at my worst. Our relationship has consistently been healthy and strong because we both work at it and care for it. We have been through good and bad times together and always lift each other up, supporting each other through all the challenges of life. This is what healthy friendship looks like.

Keep company with people that help you grow and that you enjoy spending time with. Do not bother with people who make you feel bad or tear you down in any way, shape or form. Those people are not friends. Real friends support you and lift you up.

Friends play a critical role in our lives. We learn from our friends. They show us different ways of doing things. Our friends are the people we hang out with the most. We make plans together, bounce ideas off one another, and help each other when times get tough. It is important to choose friends wisely; it is also important to be a good friend. (See Chapter Thirty - Be a Good Friend.)

Chapter Thirty

Be a Good Friend.

My dad used to tell me and my sister, "If you can count your real friends on one hand at the age of twenty-five, you're lucky." True friends are hard to come by.

How can you be a good friend? Listen. Have you ever been talking to someone and feel like, instead of listening to you, they are just waiting for their turn to talk? You are talking, and they are formulating their next few sentences instead of listening to what you are saying. There are quite a few people out there who need lessons in listening. I learned a lot about listening from your father. He is a great listener.

When your friend needs to talk, it's important that you give them your undivided attention and really listen to what they're saying. Slow down. Don't respond to them until you have had a chance to digest what they shared. Don't rush your response. In fact, you might tell your friend you want to think about it before you reply. You might not need to use any words at all!

It's OK to just be present with a friend in a time of need. We don't have to have all the answers or solutions. We can hold space for our friends when they need our love and support.

If a friend is pouring their heart out to you, remember it is not about you at that moment. They are reaching out for love and support. You provide that by simply sitting with them. Be present with them and listen.

It is easy to get consumed by our own lives. We all have daily stresses and things we need to do. Being a good friend means putting that aside for another person's benefit. Don't get so wrapped up in your own life that you forget to check in with your friends.

Be empathetic and helpful. If you've got a friend who is having trouble, put yourself in their shoes for a moment and try to help them work through the situation. Share difficult times you have gone through and describe how you managed it.

When I was struggling through your grandmother's dementia, I found it especially consoling talking to people who had also experienced the painfully slow loss of a parent to Alzheimer's disease. The patience and empathy received from those friends was particularly comforting. They listened to me when I needed to talk. I heard their stories of similar experiences and felt a connection of understanding with them. When we share these experiences, it helps us to not feel alone through the process of grief.

We may have such a strong desire to help a friend, we forget to finish listening before we start trying to fix the problem. Always remember to listen first. Listen completely. When you have the whole story, you can think through it clearly and try to help. Don't rush to fix a problem you don't thoroughly understand. First listen, then think, then speak. It may be a good idea to ask, "Do you want help? Or do you just need to talk?"

Keep in regular contact with your friends. Check in on your pals often. Call them just to say hi and see how they're doing. Text them when you think of them. Make time to hang out and do things with your friends often. (See Chapter Eleven - Nurture Your Relationships.)

Friends are the family we choose. The bonds we create with our friends can be stronger than those we share with our own flesh and blood. Take care of your friendships! Show up when no one else will. Be there in good times as well as bad. Help your friend move (this is a mark of a true-blue pal). Be a good friend and the rewards will be immeasurable.

Chapter Thirty-One

Keep an Open Mind.

Everyone does things their own way. Big stuff and little stuff - we all have our own ideas about how matters should be handled. Your Grandma Kristy told me many years ago, "There are lots of ways." My way is not necessarily right or better. If I keep an open mind, I have more opportunities to learn from others.

Human beings are diverse. We have a lot to learn from each other. People differ in what they eat, how they dress, their work, their hobbies, what music they listen to, how they worship, where they live, and the list goes on. Think of how limited our food choices would be without the influence of other cultures. How much music would we have missed out on if we were limited to only one style? What fashion trends would we have never known about? Our diversity is one of our greatest strengths and we should learn from those around us.

When we get stuck in our own way, it sends the message to others that, "I don't need you." Reacting to someone with an attitude of, "you don't know what you're doing," is hurtful and closed minded. Nobody likes to be on the receiving end of that message.

Keeping an open mind allows you to be more creative, improve your relationships and develop better problem-solving skills. Be careful not to become rigid. Listen to others. Respect their ideas and be open to new ways of doing things. Everyone benefits when we work and learn together.

There have been plenty of times in my own life that I discovered someone else's way was actually better than mine. For example, Christina taught me to cut jalapeno peppers with a plastic baggie over my hand. Before sharing this with me, I would burn my eyes every time I cut jalapenos by touching them after my hands had hot pepper juice on them. Christina's simple technique prevented me from hurting my eyes. What a shame it would be to deny myself a new and improved method.

Most of us hold our heads up a little higher when someone acknowledges we are right about something. It feels good to be right. We've all had that moment of thinking, "Ha! I was right!" We feel vindicated in these moments.

It feels better to be open and flexible. The best way we learn is by making mistakes. Thinking we are right all the time leads to rigidity, reducing our ability to learn new things. Accepting our limitations and listening to different ideas and methods opens our minds to fresh ways of thinking and learning.

Do not limit yourself by insisting on your way. When we openly welcome different ideas and processes, we grow exponentially. We become an example for those around us to follow. Don't get caught in the "my way or the highway" mentality. Allow others to teach you new things.

Chapter Thirty-Two

Don't Get Stuck in Anger or Sadness.

The day I checked my mom into the nursing home was the worst day of my life. I remember how heavy I felt, like there was a giant, wet, wool blanket on me and I could not remove it. I was losing my mother to Alzheimer's disease. I had no choice but to put her in a nursing home because I could not take care of her. Her condition was too severe, and I still had two elementary age children at home. This was the darkest time I have endured in my life.

The experience took a toll on me like nothing else ever has. I was sad beyond measure, angry at God, and I couldn't find a reason to smile for months. I tried going through the motions, mostly for you girls' sake. Every day I would force a smile, go to work, and try my best to get through the day. Truthfully, I was in the pit of depression and could not see any light or way out. It was all I could do to get out of bed in the morning during those painful days.

The breakthrough finally came one Sunday morning when your dad was preaching for us at church. He wrote the sermon for me, I am certain. It was a sermon on suffering and why we must bear it.

Your dad was able to cut through the pain and get to the source of my despair. I came to understand that we all suffer. Suffering increases our capacity for love and understanding. It is awful and painful. Nobody wants to feel it, but alas, we all do. When I realized this truth, I began healing. The situation with your grandmother never got any better, but I began dealing with my emotions in a healthier way.

My sister, Kathleen, and I worked together through the whole journey. We supported each other every step of the way. Having her with me was comforting because I knew she was dealing with the same feelings I was. We talked almost every day during that time. I am grateful we had each other to lean on.

Anger is a mask for sadness. It feels easier to be mad than to experience heartbreak. Left unchecked, anger can morph into bitterness. It is important to deal with our pain honestly. When you are feeling angry, try to figure out what is under the anger. You will usually find hurt there. The hurt is what needs to be faced and worked out.

If you find yourself sinking into depression, be sure you talk to a trusted friend or relative. When you feel sad, release your emotions. Cry. It is not fun, but it is an excellent release. When you are angry, vent. Scream. Punch something. Throw things. Do whatever helps you. Just don't get stuck.

It can be surprisingly difficult to pull yourself out of sadness, rage, or despair. Lean on your loved ones and allow them to help you. If all else fails, call your mom. I will always do whatever I can to help you.

Chapter Thirty-Three

Make Your Marriage Your Top Priority.

Your marriage will be the single most important relationship of your entire life. This life-long partnership sets the stage for everything that comes after the wedding. Do not rush into marriage.

Long before I met your father, I rushed into a marriage with another man. He was not a bad person, just not the right man for me. I was laser focused on planning the wedding, but I neglected to nurture the marriage. Once married life set in, it did not look or feel the way I had always imagined. My ex-husband and I did not do a good job of planning our future and our relationship fell apart in less than two years. Looking back, I see clearly now that neither one of us was ready for marriage.

The relationship you have with your spouse is the closest, most intimate and rewarding relationship you will ever have. It is, at the same time, complicated and challenging. Hopefully, it will be full of love and compassion most of the time. There will times when you hurt each other, misunderstand each other, and drive one another crazy. It is inevitable. We are human beings and there is no such thing as a "perfect marriage".

Before you say, "I do", be certain that you have chosen the right person. The right person will be one who accepts you exactly as you are. You'll want to spend the rest of your life with a man who treats you well and enjoys life with you. Be sure you share the same priorities with your future spouse.

Once children enter the picture, it is easy to get your priorities mixed up. The love parents have for their children is like no other love. It can feel all-consuming and even overwhelming. We want what is best for our kids and we can lose sight of the foundational relationship that came before. Be careful not to neglect your marriage when you have kids.

Your words and actions matter more than I can say. Children are keenly observant and learn from everything they see and hear around them. The example we give our kids at home is the most important example they will ever receive from anyone. This is especially true of the husband-wife relationship they witness between their parents.

When you have children, you and their father will be their first and primary teachers of how to live. If your kids grow up watching their mom and dad treat each other with love and respect, they will follow suit. Children who grow up in abusive homes often end up in abusive relationships because it's the only example they have been shown.

Just like the foundation of a home is the most crucial part of the structure, your marriage is the foundational part of your life and family. Everything is built on top of that foundation. If your marriage crumbles, everything else does too. Work on it. Keep it strong. Maintain it. Reinforce it when necessary. Cherish your marriage.

I hope that you fall in love and marry the man of your dreams one day. I hope you are both loved and adored by your future husbands and that you develop strong, healthy, unbreakable bonds. Talk through the hard stuff. (See Chapter Eleven - Nurture Your Relationships, Chapter Twenty-Eight - Be a Good Communicator, and Chapter Thirty - Be a Good Friend). Love isn't always easy, but it is worth working for.

Remember, love is a verb. It is not just an adjective or a noun. Actively love your husband as he actively loves you. Remind one another regularly that you love each other. Put each other first. The rest of your life will fall into place around your marriage. Do not let anything distract you from putting your marriage first.

Chapter Thirty-Four

Play With Your Children.

I had a difficult time with pregnancy. I miscarried several times. This created a feeling of failure inside me. I also felt pressure because I was getting older. The stress made it even harder to conceive and carry a pregnancy to term.

One of the miscarriages ended in an ectopic pregnancy. I did not know that I was carrying twins. One of them was inside one of my fallopian tubes. As a result, I had to have that fallopian tube removed and my chances of successfully conceiving were cut in half. Morgan is my miracle baby.

After Morgan was born, we tried for almost a year to conceive Christina, but again we were unsuccessful. I began to think I could not have another child. The day I discovered I was pregnant with Christina was a wonderful surprise.

Your dad and I wanted you girls desperately. I wanted to be a mom more than anything. Failing to conceive made that desire even stronger. When both of you were born, I knew that being your mom would be the most important thing I will ever do.

Raising you girls through your childhood has been the best time of my life. It wasn't easy, but it has been more rewarding than anything else I've ever done.

I loved setting up all your stuffed animals for you on the couch so you could play with them. Reading to you was one of the great delights in my life. It was not hard for either of you to convince me to read three or four books to you before bedtime. Our weekly trips to the library were super fun and I cherish those memories. All the time we spent playing at the beach or going to the park bring joyful memories to my mind. Playdates with your preschool pals and elementary school friends were enjoyed by all. I'm grateful for all the time we spent playing together.

The rewards keep coming as I see you succeeding and thriving in your own lives. I am grateful for every moment we had together and all the wonderful experiences we enjoyed while you grew up. Those years went by fast. I'm blessed and thankful that I didn't miss anything.

Based on my experience and scientific research, I encourage you to give your kids your attention as often as you possibly can. Don't miss anything. Treasure every moment with your children. It will bless you and them both.

It is hard to keep up with all the demands on us, especially during the years we are raising children. Kids are needy. They want their parents' undivided attention all the time. It is challenging to balance their needs along with work, taking care of your home, and other obligations and surprises.

Work, home, and obligations will always be there. Your children will not be in your care forever. You only get eighteen years or so.

If you are lucky enough to be able to stay home with your kids, I highly recommend it. I was willing to sacrifice my career and income in order to stay home and raise you myself. For many people, that is not financially realistic. Either way, spend quality time with your children as often as you can.

We don't get to go back and do it over again. I cannot over emphasize how important it is to recognize the value of spending time with your children when they are little. Play with them. Read to your babies. Enjoy your toddlers. Teach them and guide them. We get a short time to cherish our children before they are grown and gone.

Chapter Thirty-Five

Know Your Children's Friends.

While you were growing up, I encouraged you to have your friends over for play dates and sleepovers. This proved to be an awesome way to get to know your friends as well as their parents.

It blessed you and your friends to have a safe place to play with adequate supervision while enjoying the freedom and fun of being kids. It blessed me and your dad to provide such an environment for you and your childhood friends.

As parents, we have limited control over the crowd our kids end up in. However, establishing a relationship with your children's friends is a great way to help ensure your kids are hanging out with good people.

Your dad and I have some "not kids", as we call them. These are longtime friends of you girls that we have gotten close to. These special friends include Veronica, Iris, and Isabella as well as Maria, Ellie and Alison, Julie and Gabby. I would be remiss if I did not include Michael and Morgan's boyfriend, Gavin. It has been a joy to get to know these wonderful people and we are blessed to still call them our "not kids" even now that they are adults. We have great memories with these kids over the years and look forward to making more now that they are grown.

Be involved in your kids' lives. Talk to them about their relationships outside of the home. Ask them questions about their friends, teachers, and others they interact with regularly. Sometimes you will have to ask several ways before you get an answer. Teach them what good friendships look like and what kinds of behaviors are indicative of unhealthy relationships.

Good friends lift you up and help you in hard times. Forgiveness is an important ingredient in a healthy friendship. Anyone who puts you down or makes you feel bad about yourself is not a good friend. These are important lessons your children will take with them throughout the course of their lives. (See Chapter Thirty - Be a Good Friend.)

I recommend developing relationships with the parents of the friends your kids play with. The apple doesn't fall far from the tree. Getting to know the parents gives you more insight into the kind of people and family your children are engaging with. This insight gives you a better vantage point to advise from.

Some of my closest friendships have come out of getting to know the parents of my children's pals. During Morgan's Kindergarten year, I met two of my best buddies, Jen and Liz. When Christina entered Kindergarten, I met another great friend, Marlena. All three of these amazing moms are still among my close friends. We have enjoyed raising our kids together and supporting one another through the adventures of parenting.

Everything we did with our kids was more fun because of our friendships. Liz was Morgan's Girl Scout leader, and our friendship made the troop more fun to be a part of.

Jen and I worked together at the dance studio that both our girls attended, making every recital more enjoyable for all of us.

Marlena and I took our daughters shopping for homecoming and prom dresses together. We were Ambassa-moms when both our girls were in a singing group called "The Fenton Ambassadors" in high school. Doing these things together with our kids made all of it more fun for everyone.

Your father and I have been blessed by developing relationships with your friends. We have enjoyed making friends with the parents of your childhood pals and continue to nurture those relationships. I hope you will heed this advice and get to know your children's friends.

Chapter Thirty-Six

Take Time for Yourself.

Being a mother is a full-time job. It is the most difficult, challenging, all consuming, wonderful, and rewarding job I have ever had. While your children will be the biggest blessing in your lives, they will also drive you crazy at times. I mean, CRAZY! Kids are super demanding of your time and attention. There will be times you need to take a break. You will be a better mom for taking the pause. Do not feel guilty when it's time for mom to take a time-out. This is necessary and will benefit the whole family.

I take my role as your mom very seriously and truly give my best to you. My hope has always been that you would grow to be the amazing young women you have become. I remember times when I felt overwhelmed and exhausted. Moms are often underappreciated. There were days I felt irritable or just plain crabby during the child rearing years. This is perfectly normal and to be expected. All parents need a break from their children from time to time.

Accept your limitations and recognize when you're getting to the end of your rope. That's the time to give yourself a reprieve. If you start feeling edgy or impatient, that is a sign. It's better to take a pause in that moment than snap at one of your kids and regret it later.

Take time for yourself each day. Just a few minutes can provide calm, peace and clarity. Go outside for a few minutes. If that is not an option, lock yourself in the bathroom for a quick moment.

It is also crucially important to spend time with your spouse without the kids. Remember, your marriage is the foundation that your family is built on. (See Chapter Thirty-Three - Make Your Marriage Your Top Priority). I fondly remember a weekend trip to Traverse City with your dad shortly after Morgan was born. We missed her terribly, but the break was good for us and my mom thoroughly enjoyed her one-on-one time with her brand new grandbaby.

Don't neglect your social life during the busy time of raising your children. Hang out with your friends. Go out to lunch with a pal. Make dinner plans with other couples that you and your significant other enjoy spending time with. Go on a weekend getaway with your husband and another couple. It is OK to have Grama and Grampa take the kids for a while so you can maintain your sanity. Your children and your parents will be blessed by spending time together. It is good for kids to have relationships with trusted adults other than their parents. These multi-generational relationships are beneficial to all.

Give yourself permission to relax. You will be a better mom if you allow yourself a few minutes each day to reset. Constantly running and trying to be everything to everyone does not work. Be calm and take time for yourself.

Chapter Thirty-Seven

Make New Friends.

We have ample opportunities to connect with our peers in our school years and in college. When we enter the work force, we make new friends with our coworkers and colleagues. Hopefully, we find other outlets such as church or community involvement to create new friendship opportunities.

The truth is chances to connect with others are less frequent as we get into our golden years. We must deliberately seek those opportunities and put effort into being engaged with other people.

One of the most important lessons I taught you ladies growing up was how to make friends. This is a skill that is valuable for your entire life. Unfortunately, I have noticed that as people get older, they tend to reduce their social interactions and become secluded. This behavior is damaging to our mind and spirit.

Our brains need social interaction. Being secluded can lead to the deterioration of a person's mental and social well-being. When we spend our days alone, we are more likely to experience depression, anxiety, and cognitive decline.

I believe one of the biggest contributors to developing dementia is separation from others. My mother isolated herself after retiring, which contributed to her deteriorating cognition. Once she realized she had dementia, she became more withdrawn. She was embarrassed and didn't want people to see her mental decline.

I remember a time when your grandma went to visit her Uncle Chuck and cousins. This was early in my mother's dementia experience. When she returned home from that trip, her cognitive condition had improved markedly. It felt like she was back to her old self. She was happy to spend time with her beloved family. Happiness is the best medicine. Being with family improved her condition. When she was alone, her dementia got worse.

I stated previously that some friends are for a reason, some are for a season, and some are for a lifetime. The seasonal friends we acquire are important. We all benefit from sharing similar experiences with others who are going through the same things. This is valuable in our journey as we help each other navigate the changes of life.

Nothing transforms your life more than having children. The friends I made after you girls were born were such a blessing to me. It was during your preschool season that I started to make a lot of new friends.

My preschool mom pals and their children joined us for playdates, lunches at Pizza Hut, and so many birthday parties. We helped each other through the early years of motherhood. These friendships were an important part of your lives and my personal growth as a woman and a mother.

During your elementary school season at the Holly Academy, I made several good friends who I am still close to. It was a blessing to have other moms to enjoy all the school activities with. We supported each other and formed a little community.

Throughout our church life, I have made many close friends. Many of my church buddies have become lifelong friends as we spend time together regularly and deepen our connections.

I have met many awesome people because of your dad's involvement in the Chamber of Commerce and the Rotary. Volunteering with your father in the community is fun and we have made a lot of friends in the process.

To keep your mind healthy and happy, I strongly urge you to make new friends over the course of your life. Get yourself out there and do things you enjoy with others who enjoy the same.

Sitting on the couch watching TV is not a great way to make new friends. Scrolling on social media doesn't make any new friends either. You've got to go out into the world and purposefully engage with other people. Find a social group or club that you like. The Rotary is a great example of a club that helps build community. Churches offer opportunities for folks to connect. Senior centers host a lot of social outings.

You will be happier throughout your life if you are socially engaged. We all need people. Never stop making new friends.

Chapter Thirty-Eight

Be Kind to Everyone.

Recently, a couple of installers came to our house when we got new appliances. The two gentlemen were nice and professional. In turn, I couldn't help but extend kindness back to them. I found myself feeling a sense of comradery and even friendship with these two people I had never met. We had friendly conversation and laughed together while they worked. The simple act of treating each other with kindness and respect resulted in a wonderful experience for me and for them.

When we begin an experience with irritation or impatience, the results are very different. Think about how you feel when you are treated rudely. How do you respond when a person is impatient or irritated with you? Most of us feel hurt or angry. I get defensive when people treat me poorly.

People who work in the service industry are treated with rudeness and impatience from the customers they serve. Clients often do not have tolerance for strangers in their home, even when those strangers are doing a service the customer hired them to do.

Our words are powerful. Kind words have a positive effect on people while harsh words cause damage. We can never take our words back. Be careful with them. A thousand apologies will not erase the hurt caused by speaking callously to someone.

There are no guarantees in life. I suggest treating every conversation as if it might be the last one you have with whom it is you're talking to. What do you want your last words to that person to be? Be thoughtful about what you say to others. It matters a lot.

A little kindness goes a long way. I have found showing kindness to others blesses both the recipient and the giver in surprising ways. It is not difficult, and everyone can do it.

How does it make you feel when people are kind to you? When you are paid a compliment, what happens to your state of mind? It feels good when others show kindness to us, especially when it is unprompted. I am in a better mood after being treated nicely by other people. My improved attitude makes me more likely to show kindness to others throughout my day.

Aunt Le is one of the sweetest people on the planet. I have tried to emulate her genuine kindheartedness for my entire adult life. She makes everyone feel loved and welcome. Every time I see Aunt Le, she showers me with love and kindness. She has gone to great lengths to support people in her family as well as many of her friends. Aunt Le has given a lot of herself to help children at St. Jude Hospital and to help senior citizens in her local community. Her volunteer work for veterans is another illustration of her gentle and loving heart. Aunt LeAnn is a wonderful example to you, her adored great-nieces, and to me as well. I am ever grateful for the kindness she has shown me for my whole life.

In the hustle and bustle of everyday life, we can bless others with a simple act of kindness. You can turn someone's day around by offering a kind word or smile. The feeling you get when you treat someone nicely is one of spiritual satisfaction. It feels good to be kind to people. Kindness is contagious. When you start the kindness ball rolling, others will keep it going. Smile at people. Give compliments freely. Say hello. Open the door for the next person coming in. Be hospitable. Be kind to everyone.

Chapter Thirty-Nine

Be Brave.

Your Great Grandma Pat Morgan was an amazing woman. She was married at the tender age of sixteen. Pat had two children, Allen and my mom, Marilyn. Later, she and my grandfather adopted two more children, Greg and Debbie. Grandma Morgan was a good mom and raised all four of her children as best she could.

Your Great Grandma Pat made extra money as a seamstress. She made bride's dresses and bridesmaid's dresses for entire wedding parties. Thank God she was my grandma because she sewed all my dance costumes. Aunt Purt's and my costumes always looked better than all the other dancers because Grandma Morgan made them. Her sewing and needle work was exceptional.

My mom's dad, Gilbert Morgan, died of a heart attack when he was still in his forties. Until this time, my Grandma Morgan had never driven a car or had a regular paying job outside of the home. This was the turning point in her life and she bravely reinvented herself.

Your great grandmother put herself through driving school and got her driver's license. Your Aunt Purt and I agree she was a terrible driver. We had several frightening moments with her in the driver's seat. She was brave to get her license and we were brave to ride with her.

Next, she put herself through nursing school. Upon completion, she started working in a hospital as an RN. Grandma lived in a nice apartment in Grand Blanc and was truly a powerhouse of a woman during this time in her life.

Grandma Morgan was open to trying new things. Pat became a good bowler. She played on two or three leagues. Golf was her favorite, and she was great at it. Your Grandma Marilyn and Great Grandma Morgan were unbeatable partners at the Euchre table. I don't think your Aunt Purt and I won against them even one time! She learned a great deal because of her courageous willingness to simply try.

Your Great Grandma Morgan was not afraid of change. She bravely did what she needed to do to not only survive but live a happy and fulfilling life. The choices she made helped her through a difficult period and also improved her life drastically! She fearlessly did things that most women at that time were not doing, and moreover, were not expected to do. The older I get, the more I appreciate the example of courage and bravery your great grandmother showed me.

Taking risks in life can be scary. There are no guarantees. If we are too careful, however, we miss out on some of life's most rewarding opportunities. Do not let fear stop you from realizing your dreams. Take a chance when you have one. If I would not have taken a chance with your father, you ladies would not be here reading this book right now. Some risks are worth taking.

If you need help discerning whether a risk is worth taking, talk to a trusted friend or loved one. Pray about it. There will be times you won't have time to do either. I suggest using that gut instinct I talked about in Chapter One - Trust Your Gut.

Try not to respond to any opportunity with fear. You are capable of more than you know. Believe in yourself. You can do anything you put your mind to. Be brave.

Epilogue

My mother adored you girls. I wish she could see the amazing women you have become. I hope the stories I share about her give you a glimpse of her wisdom and the remarkable woman she was.

Your grandma was one of the smartest people I have ever known. She loved your Aunt Purt (Kathleen) and me fiercely. Her blessing to me is a blessing to you because she taught me how to be a good mom. Her wisdom shined through me all the years of your childhood.

I could have written a longer book of advice to you ladies, but I wanted to give you a guidebook to highlight the more important lessons I've learned in my own life. I hope you will refer to this book of insights often throughout your life and that it is helpful to you. There are lessons that are plain and simple while other lessons are more complex. Regardless, these tidbits of wisdom will come in handy as you go along on your journey.

It is the pleasure of my life to be your mom. I am so proud of you. Your futures are bright, and I know you will both continue to thrive and succeed. I'm happy for you and look forward to seeing how things unfold as you continue to enter adulthood.

Maybe one day I'll write a book on parenting, but I didn't want to go too far on that topic since you ladies are nowhere near motherhood yet. Still, I feel the sections on parenting are important enough to include in this compilation.

As I stated at the beginning, I love you more than any words can ever express. You are the joy of my heart.

All my love always,

Mom

Acknowledgements

In January of 2025, Pastor Dawn led our Epiphany worship service and introduced us to Star Words. She had a basket full of wooden tags, each with a different word inscribed on them. We all picked a word randomly and she asked us to keep it somewhere we could see it every day. My word was "insight", and I hung it above my kitchen sink, the place I spend the most time at home.

Initially, I wondered, what am I supposed to do with insight? Whose insight? Is it my insight, or someone else's? I had no clue as to what I was supposed to do with my Star Word. Still, there it hung every day for me to look at while doing the dishes.

As the year went on, I read insightful books and had insightful conversations with people. I thought this must be what I'm supposed to do.

It wasn't until my youngest daughter, Christina, graduated high school that something unexpected happened. The Monday after graduation, Dawn came in to work and asked me, "So, what are you going to do with your time when Nina goes to college?"

Without much hesitation, I surprisingly said out loud, "Maybe I should write a book." She asked me what I would write a book about. "Tidbits of wisdom for my girls," I replied. I thought it would be nice to write something for my children to remember me by.

Dawn encouraged me and said, "OK. I'll check back with you later." I knew she was serious, so I wrote the following note to myself on a square sticky note: "Write a book."

That was in May. By July, I had started to jot down some ideas about what I might like to say. When I finished the first draft, my intention was to print the book but only give it to my daughters.

When I asked my husband, Johnathan, to be my editor, the book started to take a turn. I had been nervous about allowing him to see what I had written. I had never written a book before, and I did not feel confident that the writing was good enough to be published. With Johnathan's editing help, I was able to improve the manuscript substantially. He encouraged me to expand most of the chapters and add personal stories.

I changed words, moved paragraphs around, and added quite a bit of content. The book started to become… well, good! I started to feel proud of my work.

Johnathan helped me to create something worthy of publishing. Believe me, the first draft was sparce and a bit boring to read. His editing was exactly what I needed to turn a mediocre manuscript into something I am proud of. I could not have succeeded in this new adventure without his help.

Dawn and Johnathan gave me a gift I never knew I wanted! That Star Word, "Insight" became a book full of insights to share with my daughters.

I did not see the big picture until I was almost finished writing. Wow! How amazing is that?

Thank you, Dawn. You have been a huge blessing to me. Your friendship and spiritual leadership have helped me to grow and succeed in ways I never dreamed of.

Thank you, Johnathan, for helping me turn this chicken scratch into a higher quality piece of writing. I could not have done this without you. Your support and love through the process have meant the world to me.

Of course, this book is for my amazing daughters, Morgan and Christina. Thank you, my beautiful Duganettes, for increasing my capacity for love. You are the joy of my life, and I love you infinitely.

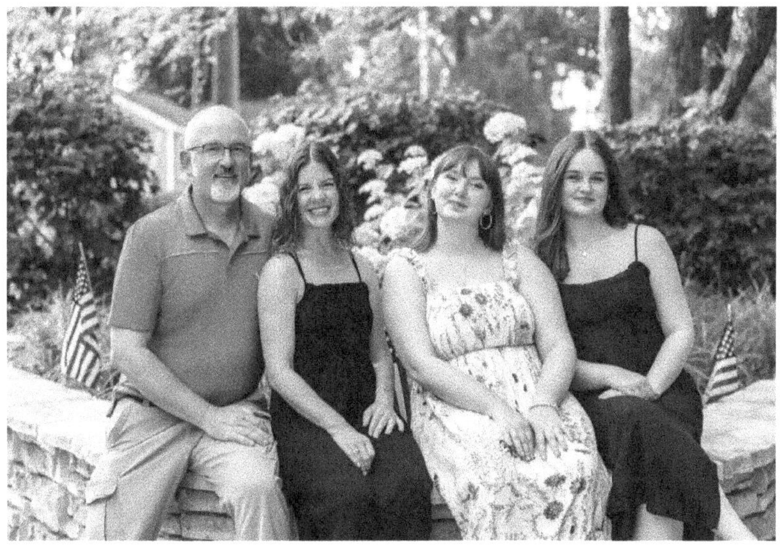

Pictured above from left to right: Johnathan, Melissa, Christina, and Morgan Dugan

Photograph by Stephanie Lane Photography

About the Author

Melissa Dugan lives with her husband, Johnathan, on Byram Lake in Linden, Michigan. Their daughter, Morgan, is a senior at the University of Michigan. Christina, their youngest, is a freshman at Michigan State University.

Melissa enjoys singing, cooking, reading, writing, exercise, and spending time with her family. Her favorite things include dinners out with family and friends and enjoying the simpler things in life. She loves a good cup of coffee and spending time in nature. Melissa's favorite event is going to see the Dave Matthews Band with her family and friends every summer.

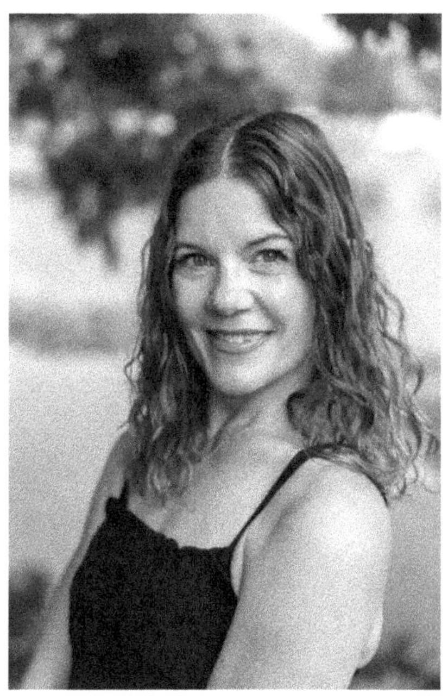

Photograph by Stephanie Lane Photography

www.ingramcontent.com/pod-product-compliance
Lightning Source LLC
LaVergne TN
LVHW010839120826
845149LV00017B/3310